MOSBY'S FUNDAMENTALS OF THERAPEUTIC MASSAGE WORKBOOK

MOSBY'S FUNDAMENTALS OF THERAPEUTIC MASSAGE WORKBOOK

Sandy Fritz
Founder, Owner, Director, and Head Instructor
Health Enrichment Center
School of Therapeutic Massage and Bodywork
Lapeer, Michigan

Kathy Paholsky, PhD
Director of Education
Health Enrichment Center
School of Therapeutic Massage and Bodywork
Lapeer, Michigan

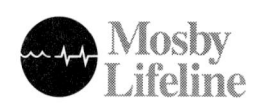

Mosby Lifeline

St. Louis Baltimore Boston Carlsbad Chicago Naples New York Philadelphia Portland
London Madrid Mexico City Singapore Sydney Tokyo Toronto Wiesbaden

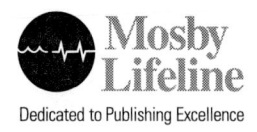

Mosby Lifeline
Dedicated to Publishing Excellence

A Times Mirror Company

Publisher: David Dusthimer
Acquisitions Editor: Eric M. Duchinsky
Assistant Editor: Christine H. Ambrose
Production Manager: Chris Baumle
Production Editor: Stacy M. Guarracino

FIRST EDITION

Copyright ©1995 by Mosby-Year Book, Inc.
A Mosby Lifeline imprint of Mosby-Year Book, Inc.

All rights reserved. No part of this publication may be reproduced, stored in a retrieval system, or transmitted, in any form or by any means, electronic, mechanical, photocopying, recording, or otherwise, without prior written permission from the publisher.

Permission to photocopy or reproduce solely for internal or personal use is permitted for libraries or other users registered with the Copyright Clearance Center, 27 Congress Street, Salem, MA 01970. This consent does not extend to other kinds of copying, such as copying for general distribution, for advertising or promotional purposes, for creating new collected works, or for resale.

Printed in the United States of America

Composition by: Mactronics, Inc.
Printing/Binding by: Plus Communications

Mosby-Year Book, Inc.
11830 Westline Industrial Drive
St. Louis, Missouri 63146

TABLE OF CONTENTS

Introduction ix

Chapter 1 : History of Massage 1
    Key Terms 1
    Puzzle 2
    Matching 3
    Time Line Exercise 4
    Problem Solving Exercise 5
    Professional Application Exercises 5
    Research For Further Study 5
    Answers 6

Chapter 2 : Professional and Legal Issues 7
    Key Terms 7
    Fill in the Blanks 9
    Puzzle 11
    Labeling 12
    Matching 13
    Additional Activities 16
    Problem Solving Exercises 17
    Professional Application 18
    Research For Further Study 18
    Answers 19

Chapter 3 : Massage and Medical Terminology 25
    Key Terms 25
    Puzzle 26
    Labeling 27
    Matching 33
    Problem Solving Exercise 34
    Professional Application 35
    Research For Further Study 35
    Answers 36

Chapter 4 : Indications and Contraindications for Massage 43
    Key Terms 43
    Fill in the Blanks 45
    Puzzle 46
    Labeling 47
    Matching 49
    Additional Activities 49
    Problem Solving Exercise 50
    Answers 51

Chapter 5 : Hygiene, Sanitation, and Safety 55
    Key Terms 55
    Fill in the Blanks 56
    Puzzle 58
    Matching 59
    Additional Activity 59
    Professional Application 60
    Answers 62

Chapter 6 : The Scientific Art 67
    Key Terms 67
    Fill in the Blanks 68
    Puzzle 70
    Labeling 71
    Matching 72
    Problem Solving Exercises 74
    Professional Application 74
    Research For Further Study 75
    Answers 76

Chapter 7 : Business and Professional Practice Management 81
    Key Terms 81
    Fill in the Blanks 82
    Puzzle 83
    Additional Activity 83
    Problem Solving Exercises 87
    Professional Application 88
    Research For Further Study 90
    Answers 91

Chapter 8 : Body Mechanics 95
    Key Terms 95
    Fill in the Blanks 96
    Labeling 97
    Additional Activity 104
    Answers 105

Chapter 9 : Getting Ready to Touch 107
    Key Terms 107
    Fill in the Blanks 108
    Puzzle 109
    Matching 110
    Additional Activity 111
    Problem Solving Exercises 112
    Professional Application 112
    Research For Further Study 113
    Answers 114

Chapter 10 : Massage Manipulations and Techniques 117
- Key Terms 117
- Fill in the Blanks 121
- Puzzle 124
- Matching 125
- Problem Solving Exercises 126
- Professional Application 126
- Answers 127

Chapter 11 : Designing the Massage 131
- Key Terms 131
- Fill in the Blanks 132
- Puzzle 134
- Matching 135
- Additional Activity 136
- Problem Solving Exercises 139
- Professional Application 140
- Research For Further Study 140
- Answers 141

Chapter 12 : Special Populations 147
- Key Terms 147
- Fill in the Blanks 148
- Puzzle 150
- Problem Solving Exercises 151
- Professional Application 152
- Research For Further Study 152
- Answers 153

Chapter 13 : Basic Therapeutic Approaches 155
- Key Terms 155
- Fill in the Blanks 156
- Puzzle 157
- Labeling 158
- Matching 159
- Additional Activity 160
- Problem Solving Exercises 161
- Professional Application 161
- Research For Further Study 161
- Answers 162

Chapter 14 : Wellness Education 165
- Key Terms 165
- Fill in the Blanks 166
- Puzzle 167
- Additional Activity 168
- Personal Application 168
- Answers 172

INTRODUCTION

A Message To The Students

This workbook was written as a companion text to Mosby's Fundamentals of Therapeutic Massage. Each chapter in that text has a corresponding chapter in this workbook. We hope to provide you with activities that help the information you learn "come alive." Many of the activities have answers that may be easily located in the text. Others require you to think things through and give your opinion. For those questions that require more in-depth thought, we present ideas that may or may not agree with your answers, but should help you see other possibilities. The professional application exercises and additional activities will help you to generate discussions with your classmates or fellow practitioners.

As instructors, we know how much easier it is to learn when you are relaxed and encouraged to be creative. You need to study both well and wisely. Some of our puzzles may challenge you, and some of them may make you smile. If you are planning on a career in a profession that encourages stress reduction in your clients, it is only fair that as a therapist you learn that as well. Massage therapy not only enhances the health and wellness of others, but touches each one of us. May it bring you the joy it has brought to both of us.

Kathy Paholsky
Sandy Fritz

CHAPTER 1

History of Massage

A. KEY TERMS

Match the term to the best definition.

1. allied health _____
2. anointing _____
3. gymnastics _____
4. lay practitioner _____

   a. Systematic body exercises.
   b. A division of medicine in which the professional receives training in a specific area of medicine to serve as a support for a physician.
   c. A person who provides massage without being trained in the medical sciences.
   d. An ancient practice of rubbing oils on the skin.

B. PUZZLE

Complete the crossword puzzle by supplying answers to the following clues.

ACROSS:

1. Established modern massage as a scientific subject for physicians
3. Nurse who formalized system of reflexology
7. Wrote a massage text used by physical therapists
9. Physician who created polarity therapy
10. Massage and physical therapy educator who wrote *Healing Massage Techniques*
12. Physiologist who developed manual lymphatic drainage
14. Current therapeutic massage researcher (2 words)
16. He developed Swedish massage
17. English physician who studied with Ling
18. A founder of modern surgery who used massage after surgery

DOWN:

1. Divided effects of massage into mechanical and reflex actions
2. Greek physician who wrote about manual medicine
4. Father of Medicine, he described medical benefits of massage
5. Worked with gate control theory of pain
6. Physician, author, and lecturer who is master synthesizer of soft tissue work
8. Ancient series of medical texts that included massage methods
10. Physician who worked with myofascial pain and trigger points
11. Popularized trigger point work, especially for general public
13. Developed transverse friction massage
16. Researchers, Drs. Jacobi and _____

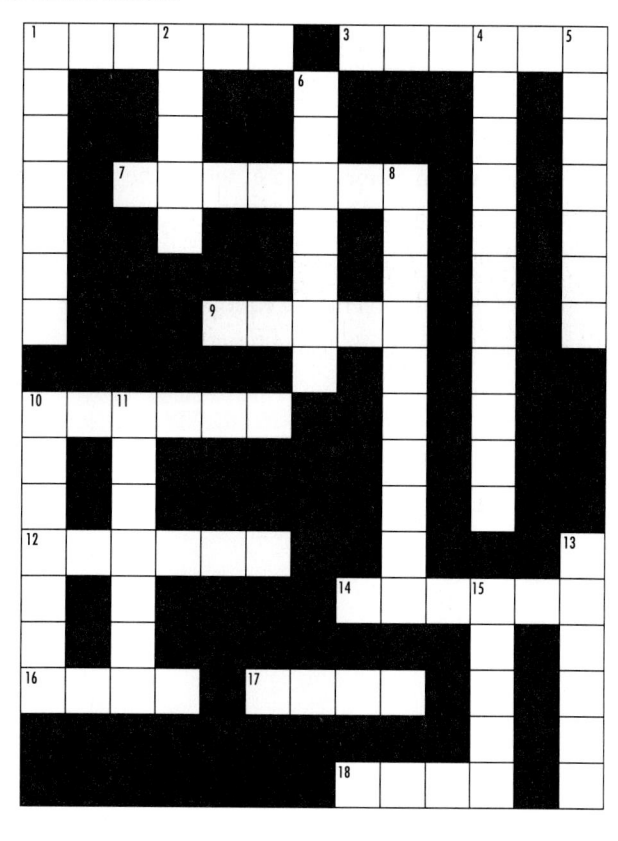

Chapter 1

C. MATCHING

Match the person or information in the first column with the most applicable response in the second column.

1. Massage in the Eastern world _____
2. Massage in the Western world _____
3. Ambrose Paré _____
4. Per Henrik Ling _____
5. Followers of Johann Mezger _____
6. Duplicated movements _____
7. Active movements _____
8. Passive movements _____
9. Charles and George Taylor _____
10. Mathias Roth _____
11. Sister Kenny _____
12. Ida Rolf _____
13. Dolores Krieger _____
14. Dr. John Harvey Kellogg _____
15. Dr. Charles Mills _____
16. Wilhelm Reich _____
17. Alexander Lowen _____
18. Elizabeth Dicke _____
19. Margaret Knott and Dorothy Voss _____
20. Esalen and Gestalt _____
21. Autonomic approach _____
22. Mechanical approach _____
23. Movement approach _____
24. Drs. Boris Chaitow and Stanley Lief _____
25. Dr. Milton Trager _____

a. called exercise
b. proposed integrated program of active and passive movements based on Swedish gymnastics
c. English physician studied with Ling
d. developed Rolfing
e. neurologist and massage advocate who criticized uneven quality of practitioners
f. founded bioenergetics
g. inspired psychotherapists to explore massage and movement therapies
h. changes abnormal movement patterns into optimal ones
i. used french terms such as *effleurage, petrissage,* etc.
j. continuation of Greco-Roman traditions
k. commonly called resistive exercise
l. co-founders of neuromuscular technique
m. developed therapeutic touch—energetic approach
n. range of motion and stretching when done by therapist
o. Battle Creek physician who used massage and hydrotherapy
p. attempts mechanical changes in soft tissue
q. introduced Swedish movements to U.S.
r. used massage for joint stiffness and wound healing after surgery
s. kept alive as part of folk culture
t. founded psychotherapeutic body techniques
u. developed Trager
v. developed connective tissue massage
w. wrote first major book on proprioceptive neuromuscular facilitation
x. used massage in polio treatment
y. exerts therapeutic effect on autonomic nervous system

D. TIME LINE EXERCISE

Place the following events, activities, and people in chronological order. The first answer is cave dweller; it is labeled number 1. Number the remaining items.

a. Art of massage first mentioned. _____
b. Ambrose Paré used massage after surgeries. _____
c. M. Leron brings Movement Cure to Russia. _____
d. Julius Caesar had himself pinched to relieve pain. _____
e. Cave dweller stubs toe and rubs it instinctively. __1__
f. Per Henrik Ling combines massage and Swedish gymnastics. _____
g. Drs. Jacobi and White research massage benefits. _____
h. Massage scandals take place in England. _____
i. Charles and George Taylor introduce Swedish movements to U.S. _____
j. Galen, an ancient Roman physician. _____
k. Albert Hoffa's text on massage published. _____
l. Polio epidemic renews interest in massage. _____
m. Connective tissue massage developed by Elizabeth Dicke. _____
n. Royal Gymnastic Central Institute established. _____
o. Celsus compiles *De Medicina*. _____
p. American Association of Masseurs and Masseuses formed. _____
q. Hippocrates encouraged physicians to use massage. _____
r. James Cyriax publishes *Textbook of Orthopedic Medicine*. _____
s. Dr. Charles Mill criticizes uneven practice of massage. _____
t. Knott and Voss write *Proprioceptive Neuromuscular Facilitation*. _____
u. National Certification Exam for Therapeutic Massage and Bodywork developed. _____

E. PROBLEM SOLVING EXERCISE

An elderly client schedules a massage. When she arrives, she relates information about a series of massage and consultation sessions she received over the years that have been beneficial to her. She cannot recall exactly what was done during these sessions, but can recall the names of the people who did the work. She wishes to know if your skills can reproduce the same success with massage she has received throughout her life. The names she provides are:

Maria Ebner, Mary McMillan, Emil Vodder, James Cyriax, Margaret Knott, Janet Travell, and Leon Chaitow.

Based on this list of professionals, list the various applications of massage and bodywork she most likely received, as well as the chapters and pages in the textbook that cover this material.

_____
_____
_____
_____

F. PROFESSIONAL APPLICATION EXERCISES

1. You are asked to present a brief lecture about the history of massage at a local historical society meeting. Develop your presentation outline. Use the lines provided for your response.

_____
_____
_____
_____
_____

2. If you were to be mentioned in a chapter on the history of massage 50 years from now, what do you imagine would be listed as your major contribution?

_____
_____
_____
_____

G. RESEARCH FOR FURTHER STUDY

Choose one professional mentioned in this history chapter. Using the reference list, recommended reading list, or other historical resources, develop an expanded list of the professional's accomplishments. Use the lines provided for your response.

_____
_____
_____
_____

ANSWERS

A. KEY TERMS
1. b
2. d
3. a
4. c

B. PUZZLE

	1M	E	2Z	G	E	R		3I	N	G	4H	A	5M
	E		A				6C				I		E
	N		L				H				P		L
	N		7D	E	S	P	A	R	8D		P		Z
	E		N				I		E		O		A
	L						T		M		C		C
	L				9S	T	O	N	E		R		K
							W		D		A		
10T	A	11P	P	A	N				I		T		
R		R							C		E		
A		U							I		S		
12V	O	D	D	E	R				N			13C	
E		D				14V	A	N	15W	H	Y		
L		E							H		R		
16L	I	N	G		17R	O	T	H			I		
									T		A		
					18P	A	R	E			X		

C. MATCHING
1. j
2. s
3. r
4. b
5. i
6. k
7. a
8. n
9. q
10. c
11. x
12. d
13. m
14. o
15. e
16. t
17. f
18. v
19. w
20. g
21. y
22. p
23. h
24. l
25. u

D. TIME LINE EXERCISE
e, a, q, d, o, j, b, f, n, c, i, g, s, h, k, l, m, p, r, t, u

E. PROBLEM SOLVING EXERCISE
Maria Ebner (connective tissue, Chapter 13, pg. 364)

Mary McMillan (therapeutic exercise with massage, Chapter 10, pg. 265)

Emil Vodder (lymphatics, Chapter 13, pg. 359)

James Cyriax (friction, Chapter 13, pg. 364)

Margaret Knott (proprioceptive neuromuscular facilitation, Chapter 10, pg. 268)

Janet Travell (trigger points, Chapter 13, pg. 368)

Leon Chaitow (neuromuscular approaches, Chapter 10, pg. 269)

CHAPTER 2

Professional and Legal Issues

A. KEY TERMS

Match the term to the best definition.

1. applied kinesiology _____
2. bodywork _____
3. boundary _____
4. certification _____
5. coalition _____
6. cranial-sacral and myofascial approaches _____
7. credential _____
8. disclosure _____
9. energetic approaches _____
10. essential touch _____
11. ethics _____
12. exemption _____
13. informed consent _____
14. integrated approaches _____
15. intimacy _____
16. license _____
17. manual lymph drainage _____
18. medical rehabilitative massage _____
19. neuromuscular approaches _____
20. oriental approaches _____
21. right of refusal _____
22. safe touch _____
23. sexual misconduct _____
24. scope of practice _____
25. structural and postural integration approaches _____
26. therapeutic massage _____
27. wellness personal service massage _____

a. Term describing all of the various forms of massage, movement, and other touch therapies.
b. Methods of bodywork that work with subtle body responses.
c. Vital, fundamental, primary touch crucial to well being.
d. Voluntary credentialing process usually requiring education and testing, administered either privately or by government regulatory bodies.

e. A tender, familiar, and understanding experience between beings.

f. Designation earned by completing a process that verifies a certain level of expertise in a given skill.

g. Standards, ideals, morals, values, and principles of honorable, decent, fair, responsible, and proper conduct.

h. Methods of bodywork that influence lymphatic movement.

i. Methods of bodywork that have developed from the ancient Chinese.

j. Methods of bodywork that influence the reflexive responses of the nervous system and its connection to muscular function.

k. Any behavior that is sexually oriented in the professional setting.

l. The where, when, and how a professional may provide a service or function as a professional.

m. Methods of bodywork derived from biomechanics, postural alignment, and the importance of the connective tissue structures.

n. Personal space located within an arms'-length perimeter. Personal emotional space designated by morals, values, and experience.

o. Combined methods of various forms of massage and bodywork styles.

p. A situation in which a professional is not required to comply with an existing law because of educational or professional standing.

q. Acknowledging and informing the client of any situation that interferes with or impacts upon the professional relationship.

r. The scientific art and system of assessment, and manual application to the superficial soft tissue of skin, muscles, tendons, ligaments, fascia, and the structures that lie in the superficial tissue using the hand, foot, knee, arm, elbow, and forearm through the systematic external application of touch, stroking (effleurage), friction, vibration, percussion, kneading (petrissage), stretching, compression, passive and active joint movements within the normal physiological range of motion, and adjunctive external applications of water, heat, and cold.

s. Methods of evaluation and adaptation that use an application of muscle testing along with various forms of massage and bodywork for corrective procedures.

t. Secure, respectful, considerate, sensitive, responsive, sympathetic, understanding, supportive, and empathetic contact.

u. The level of professional responsibility based on extensive education that prepares the massage therapist to develop, maintain, rehabilitate, or augment physical function, relieve or prevent physical dysfunction and pain, and to enhance the well being of the client. Methods include assessment of the soft tissue and joints, and treatment by soft tissue manipulation, hydrotherapy, remedial exercise programs, actinotherapy (light), and client self-care programs.

v. A type of credential required by law to regulate the practice of a profession to protect the public health, safety, and welfare.

w. Client authorization for any service from a professional, based on adequate information provided by the massage professional so that the client can make an educated choice.

x. A non-specific approach to massage with a focus on the assessment procedures to determine contraindications to massage, the need for referral to other health care professionals, and the development of a health enhancing, physical state for the client.

y. A group formed for a particular purpose.

z. Methods of bodywork that work both reflexively and mechanically with the fascial network of the body.

aa. The entitlement of both the client and the professional to stop the session.

B. FILL IN THE BLANKS

By carefully examining any style or system of massage or bodywork, one can see that some basic ideas are being used to stimulate sensory receptors, which disrupt an existing pattern in the central nervous system control centers and result in a shift in motor impulses to re-establish _____ (reflexive methods). The very same methods can be applied in a different way to change the consistency or position of connective tissue or to shift pressure in the vessel to facilitate blood and _____ (mechanical methods).

Oriental (Asian) approaches come from original _____ concepts. These _____ manipulations and stretches elicit responses in the nervous and the circulatory systems. The effects are both reflexive and mechanical. Structural and postural integration approaches focus more specifically on the connective tissue structure to influence _____ and _____. Neuromuscular approaches are of a _____ or reflexive variety. Observation of the systems reveals that connective tissue is also being affected. The common thread throughout all of the styles is the basic concepts of activation of the tonus receptor mechanism, reflex arc stimulation, positional receptors, and applications of _____.

Manual lymphatic drainage utilizes the anatomy and physiology of the mechanism of lymphatic movement with both mechanical and reflexive techniques to _____ lymphatic fluid flow. Variations of this system exist and are sometimes called _____ massage. Energetic approaches are based on ancient concepts of the body energy patterns and use _____ touch to initiate _____ responses. Cranial-sacral and myofascial approaches focus more specifically on the various aspects of both mechanical and reflexive _____ tissue functions and the concept of minute movement of the cranium and the _____. Both light and deep touch are used, depending on the method. Dr. James Cyriax's _____ methods fall into this category.

Applied kinesiology uses a specific muscle testing procedure for _____ purposes. Some of the _____ measures use Asian meridians and acupressure while others rely on the osteopathic reflex mechanisms. Integrated approaches incorporate _____ styles of bodywork, focused toward a _____ population, and are _____ of methods rather than a physiologic intervention. The expanding styles of _____ approaches to massage and bodywork are the same concepts that focus on the homeostatic balance of the autonomic nervous system, the limbic system, and the endocrine responses.

Clients have the right to refuse the massage practitioner's services. This is called the _____. It is a client's right to refuse or stop treatment at anytime. When this request is made during treatment, the therapist will _____, despite prior consent. A massage therapist has the right to refuse to treat any area of the body of a client, or to terminate the professional relationship, if the therapist feels the client is _____ the relationship. At the same time, massage therapists are bound by a _____ code of conduct. You may refuse to work with anyone, as long as you explain the reasons why. This is called _____. Be very honest with the client. When explaining the situation to the prospective client, leave out all of the _____ of the story.

A _____ is the personal space located within an arms'-length perimeter. It is also the personal emotional space designated by morals, values, and experience. We may offend someone because of differences within our _____ system. If it is too difficult for us to respect the client's boundary needs, then _____ him or her to a better-suited massage practitioner.

_____ means that client's information is private and belongs to the client. It is _____ for the massage professional to discuss anything about a client with anyone other than the client, including the client's health care professional, without the client's permission. Confidentiality is a _____.

Remember, it is the intention of the touch that is the determining factor. The touch of the massage therapist is not focused toward _____ arousal and release. The physiologic aspect of this topic is another matter. Here the therapist can set the stage and monitor _____. Keep _____ light. Change the _____. This is where the _____ skills of the practitioner come into play. The moment of _____ must be dealt with very carefully. Clients may look to the therapist for emotional support beyond the _____ scope of practice for massage. Encourage them to find the support they require from another source. If a client needs help with coping skills, _____ them to someone who is qualified to help.

The touch of a massage therapist is a _____. Safe is the ability to maintain _____ in a situation and fluctuate easily between responses to cope resourcefully with inevitable change and demands in everyday life. The therapist must consider anything, including personal beliefs and fears, that may make touch _____ for clients. By dealing with personal intimacy issues, not only can the massage therapist provide _____ touch for the client, but the client becomes able to establish proper _____. It must always be kept in mind that each individual therapist represents the_____ massage therapy profession. Demonstration of _____ for the self demonstrates respect for the profession as a whole. When ethical dilemmas are difficult to resolve, massage therapists are expected to engage in a _____ decision-making process that is explicit enough to bear public scrutiny.

The types of legislative controls most often encountered are _____ or provincial control and _____ control. States make laws that are developed to _____ the public safety and welfare. The scope of practice, or what the professional is allowed to do, is described in the law that governs the _____ professional. Local laws, usually called _____, are in place to protect the public safety and welfare.

The local government does regulate where the professional may work. This is done through _____ laws. Local governments need to establish that the massage business is legitimate therapeutic massage and not a front for prostitution. State governments have to protect the public's health, safety, and welfare from the unregulated practice of massage.

Both units of government need to protect the public from potentially dangerous acts by defining performance criteria based on _____ or the ability to pass a test. Licensing, compliance with ordinances, and passing any of the nationally recognized certification exams is _____ in the professional practice of massage. If a difficult state law or local ordinance is encountered, massage therapists must work together to _____ the regulation.

_____ means the right of exchange of privileges between governing bodies. Some states have _____ licensing requirements for professionals. When this happens, a state may _____ a different state's license. This is _____ common for many professionals, and it is even less common for massage therapists. Individual state licensing or any type of certification _____ secure the right to practice massage in any other location, other than that of the government issuing the license.

C. PUZZLE

Find the following words in the word search.

- bodywork
- boundary
- coalition
- cranial
- credential
- disclosure
- ethics
- exemption
- informed consent
- intimacy
- license
- manual lymph drainage
- massage
- medical
- neuromuscular
- ordinance
- refusal
- right
- sacral
- safe touch
- scope
- sexual misconduct
- therapeutic

```
M J O Y C I T U E P A R E H T
A S T M S A C R A L G B P N C
N C E Y F Q R J K L P M E T U
U O P I K B A R E F U S A L D
A R Y R A D N U O B N R J J N
L D E X Y G I L R O P A C E O
L I S Q R S A B C D E L R R C
Y N C H I J L D O Y B U E U S
M A O E T S E R A W O C D S I
P N P J N M O Z L O Y S E O M
H C E B R S Y M I R Y U N L L
D E C O Y X E E T K C M T C A
R T F V W D G X I Z A O I S U
A N B D I A F S O Y M R A I X
I P Q C S R C M N H I U L D E
N O A S K I H C U O T E F A S
A L A Z H G O S T X N N L I X
G M D T L H J B E A I R T U C
E X E M P T I O N L M N O P W
```

D. LABELING

Label the drawing of the Bodywork Tree, using the following words:

Reflexology, Chakras, Myofascial release, Bioenergies, Mind, Subtle energy healing, Infant massage, Reeducation movement, Muscle energy, Craniosacral

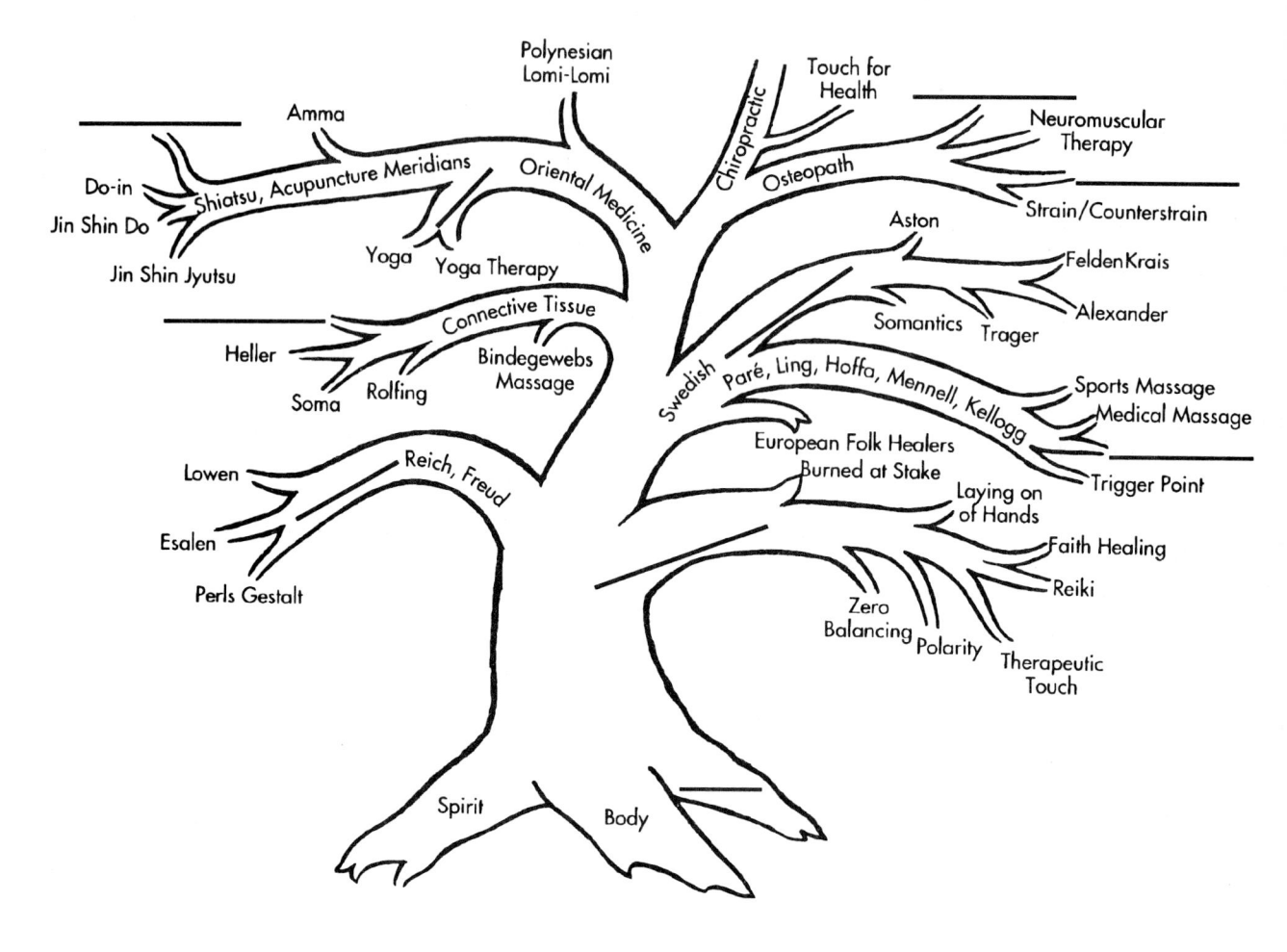

Fig. 2.1

E. MATCHING

1. Match the specific individual systems of bodywork with the basic approach and concept. Some answers will be used more than once.

1. Tuina _____
2. PNF _____
3. Vodder lymphatic drain _____
4. Rolfing _____
5. Touch for Health _____
6. Reiki _____
7. Reflexology _____
8. On-site massage _____
9. Orthobionomy _____
10. Polarity _____
11. Prenatal _____
12. Myofascial release _____
13. Deep tissue massage _____
14. Acupressure _____
15. Sports massage _____
16. Soma _____

a. Oriental
b. Structural and postural integration
c. Neuromuscular
d. Energetic approach
e. Cranial-sacral and myofascial
f. Manual lymphatic drainage
g. Applied kinesiology
h. Integrated approaches

2. *Match each profession with its appropriate scope of practice.*

1. Chiropractic _____
2. Dentistry _____
3. Medicine _____
4. Nursing _____
5. Osteopathic medicine _____
6. Physical therapy _____
7. Podiatric medicine _____
8. Psychology _____
9. Cosmetology _____
10. Medical rehabilitative massage _____
11. Therapeutic massage _____
12. Wellness personal service massage _____

a. A health-enhancing, nonspecific approach to massage for generalized stress reduction, providing benefits similar to exercise or other relaxation methods produced by massage to increase the well-being of the client. Requires approximately 500 hours of education. Supervision or consultation by a health care professional is not required.

b. A system of assessment of, and manual application to, the superficial soft tissues for the purposes of establishing and maintaining good physical condition and health and requiring approximately 1000 hours of education. With consultation or supervision from health care professionals.

c. The discipline within the healing arts that deals with the nervous system and its relationship to the spinal column and its interrelationship with the other body systems.

d. The diagnosis, treatment, prescription, or operation for a physical condition of the human tooth, alveolar process, gums, jaws, or their dependent tissues.

e. Bodywork approach supervised by a health care professional as part of a multi-disciplinary health care team dealing with illness and trauma recovery and treatment, and requiring approximately 2000 hours of education.

f. A service provided to enhance the health condition and appearance of the skin, hair, and nails. Any external preparations intended to cleanse and beautify the skin, hair, or other part of the body.

g. The diagnosis, treatment, prevention, cure, or relieving of human disease, ailment, defect, complaint, or other physical or mental condition, by attendance, advice, device, diagnostic test, or other means.

h. The systematic application of substantial specialized knowledge and skill, derived from the biological, physical, and behavioral sciences to the care, treatment, counsel, and health teachings of individuals who are experiencing changes in the normal health process or who require assistance in the maintenance of health and in the prevention or management of illness, injury, or disability.

i. The examination, diagnosis, and treatment of abnormal nails, superficial excrescences (abnormal outgrowths or enlargements) occurring on the human hands and feet.

j. The application of principles, methods, and procedures of understanding, predicting, and influencing behavior for the purposes of the diagnosis, assessment related to diagnosis, prevention, amelioration (improvement), or treatment of mental or emotional disorders, disabilities, or behavioral adjustment problems by means of psychotherapy, counseling, behavior modification, hypnosis, biofeedback techniques, psychological tests, or other verbal or behavioral means.

k. An independent school of medicine and surgery utilizing full methods of diagnosis and treatment in physical and mental health and disease, and placing special emphasis on the interrelationship of the musculoskeletal system to other body systems.

l. The evaluation or treatment of an individual by the employment of effective properties of physical measures and the use of therapeutic exercise and rehabilitative procedures with or without devices for the purposes of preventing, correcting, or alleviating a physical or mental disability. Physical measures include massage, mobilization, heat, cold, air, light, water, electricity, and sound.

3. Match the credentialing concerns with the statements to which they apply.

a. Licensing
b. Government Certification
c. Government Registration
d. Exemption
e. Professional Private Certification

1. Is voluntary, but would be required by anyone using the protected title, i.e., massage therapist. Other people can provide the service, but cannot call themselves massage therapists. _____
2. Practitioners who meet specified educational requirements could be exempt from meeting current regulatory requirements. _____
3. Requires a state or provincial board of examiners. _____
4. Requires specific educational requirements and/or examination. _____
5. Legally defines and limits the scope of practice for a profession. _____
6. Does not provide title protection. _____
7. Only valid insofar as a level of professional achievement is indicated. _____
8. Voluntary, privately administered exam. _____
9. Is voluntary. _____
10. Not required to comply with an existing regulation, either state or local. _____
11. Administered by the State Department of Registry or other appropriate state agency. _____
12. Requires everyone in the jurisdiction who practices the profession to be licensed. _____
13. Does not necessarily require specific education such as a school diploma. Often, other forms of verification of professional standards such as years in practice are acceptable. _____
14. A private type of credential. _____
15. Administered by an independent board. _____

F. ADDITIONAL ACTIVITIES

1. Standards of Practice guidelines

Label with an X those situations in which a person is not able to provide informed consent.

a. ____ Elderly client living alone
b. ____ Fifty-year-old man taking high blood pressure medication
c. ____ Freshman high school student
d. ____ Closed-head injured 30-year-old female who communicates with computer
e. ____ Twenty-four-year old developmentally disabled client
f. ____ Client who does not speak English and no interpreter is present
g. ____ Client who seems under the influence of alcohol
h. ____ Twenty-year-old woman in the third trimester of pregnancy
i. ____ Severely depressed client
j. ____ Elderly client with dementia
k. ____ Client who insists that you cure her sore knee
l. ____ Terminally ill hospice client

2. List 10 behaviors that constitute sexual impropriety or sexual abuse.

1. _____
2. _____
3. _____
4. _____
5. _____
6. _____
7. _____
8. _____
9. _____
10. _____

3. List 10 ways to maintain professional space.

1. _____
2. _____
3. _____
4. _____

5. _____
6. _____
7. _____
8. _____
9. _____
10. _____

4. *List the five steps in determining licensing needs.*

1. _____
2. _____
3. _____
4. _____
5. _____

G. PROBLEM SOLVING EXERCISES

1. A new client presents information to you concerning treatment received during a massage in another community. Some of the information seems to conflict with the principles of the code of ethics presented in your text. The client explains that the massage professional told him he needed to lose weight, did not stop working on his feet when asked to, did not explain that a trigger point area could be sore the next day, gave him a hug at the end of the session without asking first, told a joke containing sexual innuendo, let the drape slip while massaging his buttocks, talked about difficulties with her own children, walked in to get a chart without knocking first and interrupted him getting dressed after the massage, mentioned how bad physical therapists are at dealing with neck pain and that she could fix his neck problem. He also indicated that the massage professional did not give him a receipt when he paid for the massage.

   What areas of the code of ethics did the massage professional breach and how would you explain how you operate differently?

   _____
   _____
   _____
   _____

2. The following case scenarios detail situations in explaining intimacy issues. After reading each situation, write down two or three ways to deal with the issue. Three different responses will be provided for you to compare with your answers.

   A. Kathy has been a massage professional for three years. She has been seeing Mr. Adams for a monthly massage for two years. He is in the process of a divorce and begins to schedule a massage every week because of the stress he is under. Last week he mentioned to Kathy how important the massage is for him and lightly touched her hand. Should Kathy be concerned? List three options for dealing with the issue.

B. Massage therapist Mat has been a massage professional for 10 years. Just recently he has been seeing a client named Jeff who attended the same high school that he did. While they were only acquaintances during school, Jeff speaks often of the good old school days. At the last appointment, Jeff offered an extra hockey game ticket to Mat and asked if he would like to go with him. List three options for dealing with the issue.

C. Mary is new to the massage therapy profession. She has only had a few clients. She finds a new client very attractive and notices that she is spending extra time with that client each session. She recognizes that she is attracted to the client physically and emotionally. List three options for dealing with the issue.

H. PROFESSIONAL APPLICATION

You are relocating to a state different from where you received your massage education and need to locate information concerning regulatory requirements to practice. What are your resources and what government agencies do you need to contact?

I. RESEARCH FOR FURTHER STUDY

Choose a profession and trace its professional development. Correlate its progress with the professional development of therapeutic massage.

ANSWERS

A. KEY TERMS

1. s
2. a
3. n
4. d
5. y
6. z
7. f
8. q
9. b
10. c
11. g
12. p
13. w
14. o
15. e
16. v
17. h
18. u
19. j
20. i
21. aa
22. t
23. k
24. l
25. m
26. r
27. x

B. FILL IN THE BLANKS (answers appear in order of occurrence in text)

homeostasis
lymph circulation

Chinese
compressive
posture
biomechanics
nervous
stretch and lengthening

stimulate
systemic
light
reflexive
connective
dura
cross-fiber friction

evaluation
corrective
many
specific
combinations
body and mind

right of refusal
comply
sexualizing
nondiscrimination
disclosure
details

boundary
value
refer

Confidentiality
unethical
trust

sexual
responses
discussions
topic
interpersonal
intimacy
ethical
refer

safe touch
well being
unsafe
essential
boundaries
entire
respect
conscientious

state
local
protect
licensed
ordinances

zoning

education
important
change

Reciprocity
similar
accept
not
does not

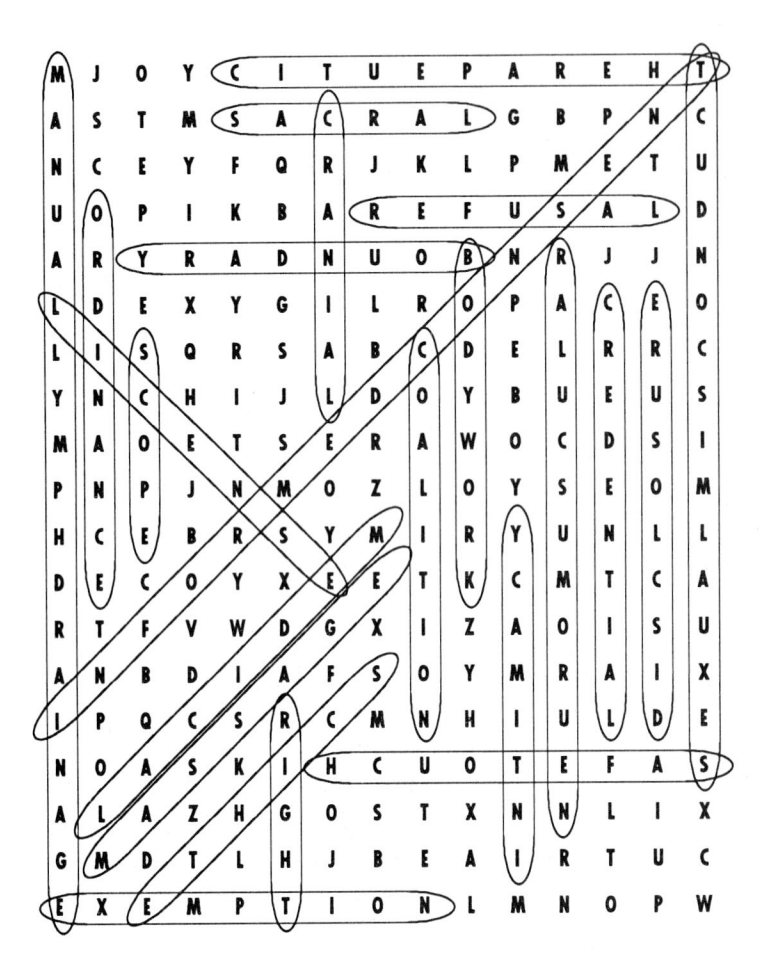

C. PUZZLE

M	J	O	Y	C	I	T	U	E	P	A	R	E	H	T
A	S	T	M	S	A	C	R	A	L	G	B	P	N	C
N	C	E	Y	F	Q	R	J	K	L	P	M	E	T	U
U	O	P	I	K	B	A	R	E	F	U	S	A	L	D
A	R	Y	R	A	D	N	U	O	B	N	R	J	J	N
L	D	E	X	Y	G	I	L	R	O	P	A	C	E	O
L	I	S	Q	R	S	A	B	C	D	E	L	R	R	C
Y	N	C	H	I	J	L	D	O	Y	B	U	E	U	S
M	A	O	E	T	S	E	R	A	W	O	C	D	S	I
P	N	P	J	N	M	O	Z	L	O	Y	S	E	O	M
H	C	E	B	R	S	Y	M	I	R	U	E	N	L	L
D	E	C	O	Y	X	E	E	T	K	C	M	T	C	A
R	T	F	V	W	D	G	X	I	Z	A	O	I	I	U
A	N	B	D	I	A	F	S	O	Y	M	R	A	X	X
I	P	Q	C	S	R	C	M	N	H	I	U	L	D	E
N	O	A	S	K	I	H	C	U	O	T	E	F	A	S
A	L	A	Z	H	G	O	S	T	X	N	N	L	I	X
G	M	D	T	L	H	J	B	E	A	I	R	T	U	C
E	X	E	M	P	T	I	O	N	L	M	N	O	P	W

D. LABELING

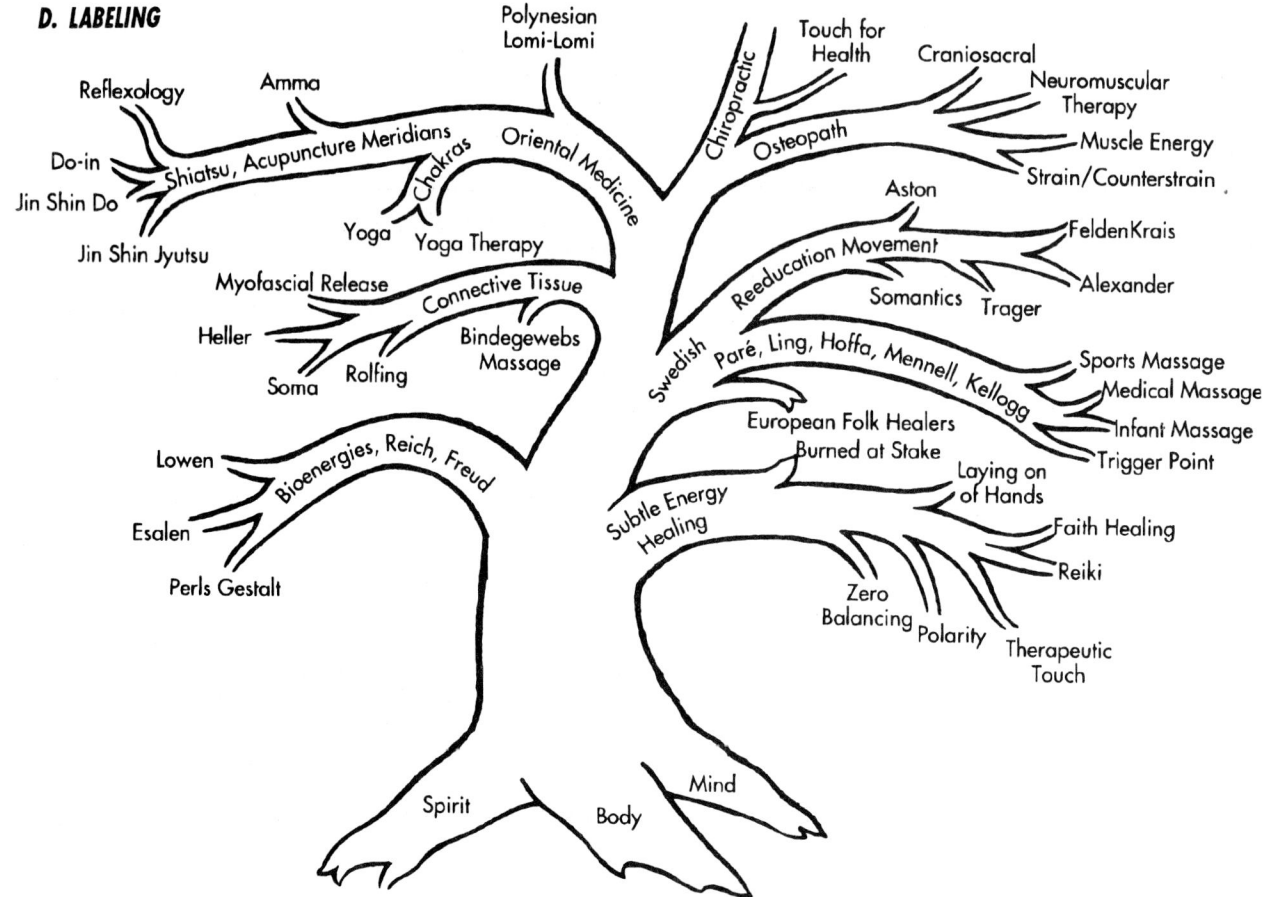

Tree diagram labels:

Reflexology, Amma, Polynesian Lomi-Lomi, Touch for Health, Craniosacral, Neuromuscular Therapy, Do-in, Shiatsu, Acupuncture Meridians, Chiropractic, Muscle Energy, Jin Shin Do, Chakras, Oriental Medicine, Osteopath, Strain/Counterstrain, Jin Shin Jyutsu, Yoga, Yoga Therapy, Aston, FeldenKrais, Myofascial Release, Reeducation Movement, Alexander, Heller, Connective Tissue, Somantics, Trager, Soma, Rolfing, Bindegewebs Massage, Swedish, Paré, Ling, Hoffa, Mennell, Kellogg, Sports Massage, Medical Massage, European Folk Healers Burned at Stake, Infant Massage, Lowen, Bioenergies, Reich, Freud, Laying on of Hands, Trigger Point, Esalen, Subtle Energy Healing, Faith Healing, Perls Gestalt, Reiki, Zero Balancing, Polarity, Therapeutic Touch

Spirit, Body, Mind

Chapter 2

E. MATCHING

1. Match the specific individual systems of bodywork with the basic approach and concept.

1. a
2. c
3. f
4. b
5. g
6. d
7. c
8. h
9. c
10. d
11. h
12. e
13. e
14. a
15. h
16. b

2. Match each profession with its appropriate scope of practice.

1. c
2. d
3. g
4. h
5. k
6. l
7. i
8. j
9. f
10. e
11. b
12. a

3. Match the credentialing concerns with the statements to which they apply.

1. b
2. d
3. a
4. a
5. a
6. c or d
7. e
8. e
9. c or e
10. d
11. c
12. a
13. c
14. e
15. b

F. ADDITIONAL ACTIVITIES

1. c, e, f, g, i, j, k

2. List 10 behaviors that constitute sexual impropriety or sexual abuse.

The therapist dating a client.
Disrobing or draping practices that reflect a lack of respect for the client's privacy.
Deliberately watching a client dress or undress.
Sexual comments about a client's body or underclothing.
Making sexualized or sexually demeaning comments to a client.
Criticism of the client's sexual orientation.
Discussion of the potential sexual performance.
Conversations regarding the sexual preferences or fantasies of the client or the massage therapist.
Requests to date.
Kissing of a sexual nature.
Genital to genital contact.
Oral to genital contact.
Oral to anal contact.
Oral to oral contact (except CPR).
Oral to breast contact.
Touching or undraping the genitals, perineum, or anus.
Touching or undraping breasts.
Encouraging the client to masturbate in the presence of the massage therapist.
Masturbation by the massage therapist while the client is present.
Masturbation of the client by the massage therapist.

3. List 10 ways to maintain professional space.

Keep a picture of family members in the reception area or the therapy room.
Share a little of the family background.
Wear a uniform or maintain a style of dress that is professional and different from casual clothes.
Use an answering machine or service, receptionist or secretary, and return calls within set hours.
Maintain regular appointment hours.
Begin and end sessions on time.
Do not spend personal time, such as lunch, etc., with clients.
Record client policies and rules clearly and concisely, and make sure that the client reads them.

Post client policies and rules on the wall to provide additional reinforcement.

Educate clients by answering their questions intelligently, based on physiology.

Never work behind a locked door.

4. List the five steps in determining licensing needs.

1. Find out if your state or provincial requires licensing. If state licensing exists, then find out what the educational requirements are to sit for the boards.

2. If your state does not have licensing, contact the local government where you intend to work to see if there is a local ordinance.

3. Contact the State Department of Education and confirm that the school you plan to attend is licensed and in compliance with state regulations.

4. Contact the local government concerning zoning requirements and building codes.

5. Contact the local government and apply for any permits or business licenses required.

G. PROBLEM SOLVING EXERCISES

1. (Numbers mentioned are the code of ethics numbers from the text.)

The client explains that the massage professional:

told him he needed to lose weight, 1

did not stop working on his feet when asked to, 11

did not explain that a trigger point area could be sore the next day, 10

gave him a hug at the end of the session without asking first, 9

told a joke containing sexual innuendo, 18

let the drape slip when massaging the buttocks, 11

talked about difficulties with her children, 22

walked in to get a chart without knocking first and interrupted him getting dressed after the massage, 1

mentioned how bad physical therapists are at dealing with neck pain and that she could fix it, 3 and 8

no receipt was given for his payment, 14.

2. A.

1. Ignore the situation and see if it occurs again.

2. After the massage, when both are in the office area, talk with Mr. Adams about how she understands the extra stress he is under, but it is important to remember the boundaries of the therapeutic relationship. During times of loss it is easy to personalize a professional relationship. (Transference)

3. Acknowledge the touch at the time it happens and gently explain that while she understands that the massage helps with the stress and provides for professional companionship it is important for both to remember the ethical standards of massage and the professional relationship.

2. B.

1. Thank Jeff for the ticket but refuse, explaining the importance of not spending time with clients outside the professional setting, even with a past acquaintance.

2. Talk with Jeff after the massage and explain that while it is pleasant to remember school days, being a professional providing massage services and spending social time together doesn't mix. Thank him for the ticket but refuse to accept.

3. Let Jeff know that if you accept the ticket, then the professional relationship will have to end, and he can see another therapist at the same office from now on.

2. C.

1. Mary could acknowledge that her feelings are a form of countertransference and have nothing to do with the client, restore the professional boundaries and time limits of the massage, and continue to see the client.

2. Mary can speak with the client about her feelings in a very brief way, explaining the difficulty with maintaining the professional relationship, and refer the client to another therapist.

3. Mary can initiate peer review by talking to an experienced therapist. Another massage professional can understand the interactions that take place in the therapy room, and may be able to give her some good recommendations as to how to handle such a situation. Using this peer support system is an excellent method of preserving our professional integrity, and providing encouragement and guidance for each other.

H. PROFESSIONAL APPLICATION

Resources: Professional organization, state licensed schools, practicing massage professionals

Government agencies: State department of licensing and regulation, Local government officials

CHAPTER 3

Massage and Medical Terminology

A. KEY TERMS

Match the term to the best definition.

1. abbreviation _____
2. combining vowel _____
3. prefix _____
4. root _____
5. suffix _____
6. word element _____

   a. A vowel added between two roots or a root and a suffix to facilitate pronunciation.
   b. Word element comprising the fundamental meaning of the word.
   c. A word element placed at the beginning of a word to alter the meaning of the word.
   d. A reduced form of a word or phrase.
   e. A part of a word.
   f. A word element placed at the end of a root to alter the meaning of the word.

B. PUZZLE

This is a game that uses a special code. Key words from this chapter have been "translated" into a different alphabet. Once you find what one letter stands for, use that code for this entire puzzle.

The first word is given to you to help you get started.

1. qdywkmek — anterior

So, in this puzzle, q stands for a, d stands for n, y stands for t, w stands for e, and so on.

2. zqxlnu
3. sxqdyqk
4. kwrnbfwdy
5. imuyqx
6. bwimqx
7. swkmspwkqx
8. zexqk
9. wkwry
10. unsmdw
11. mdcwkmek
12. skejmbqx
13. iekuqx
14. xqywkqx
15. unswkcmrmqx

C. LABELING

Label the directions and planes of the body for Figure 3.1.

A. superior/cranial
B. anterior/ventral
C. inferior/caudal
D. posterior/dorsal
E. frontal plane
F. sagittal plane
G. transverse plane

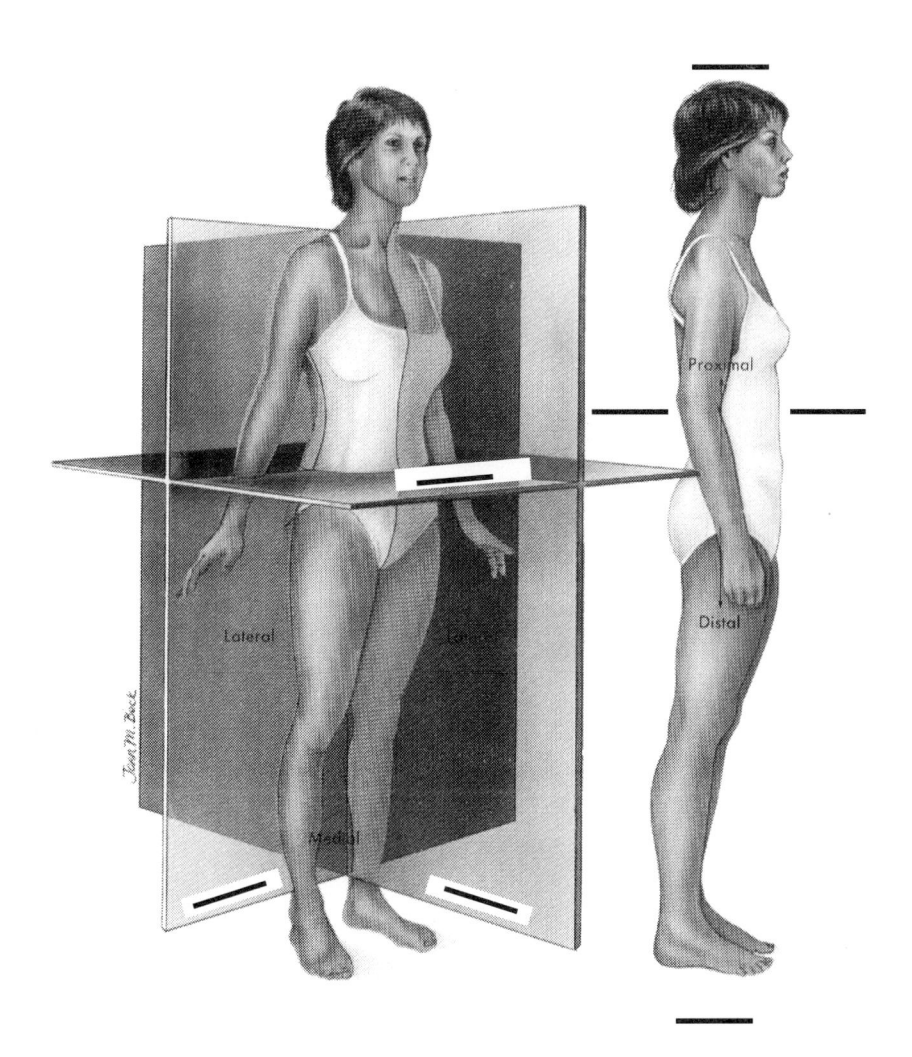

Fig. 3.1

Label the skeletal system for Figure 3.2A that shows the anterior view of the skeleton.

a. cranium
b. nasal bone
c. maxilla
d. mandible
e. orbit
f. clavicle
g. sternum
h. xiphoid process
i. costal cartilage
j. ilium
k. pubis
l. ischium
m. carpals
n. metacarpals
o. phalanges
p. sacrum
q. greater trochanter
r. coccyx
s. lesser trochanter
t. femur
u. patella
v. tibia
w. fibula
x. tarsals
y. metatarsals
z. phalanges
aa. humerus
bb. vertebral column
cc. ulna
dd. radius

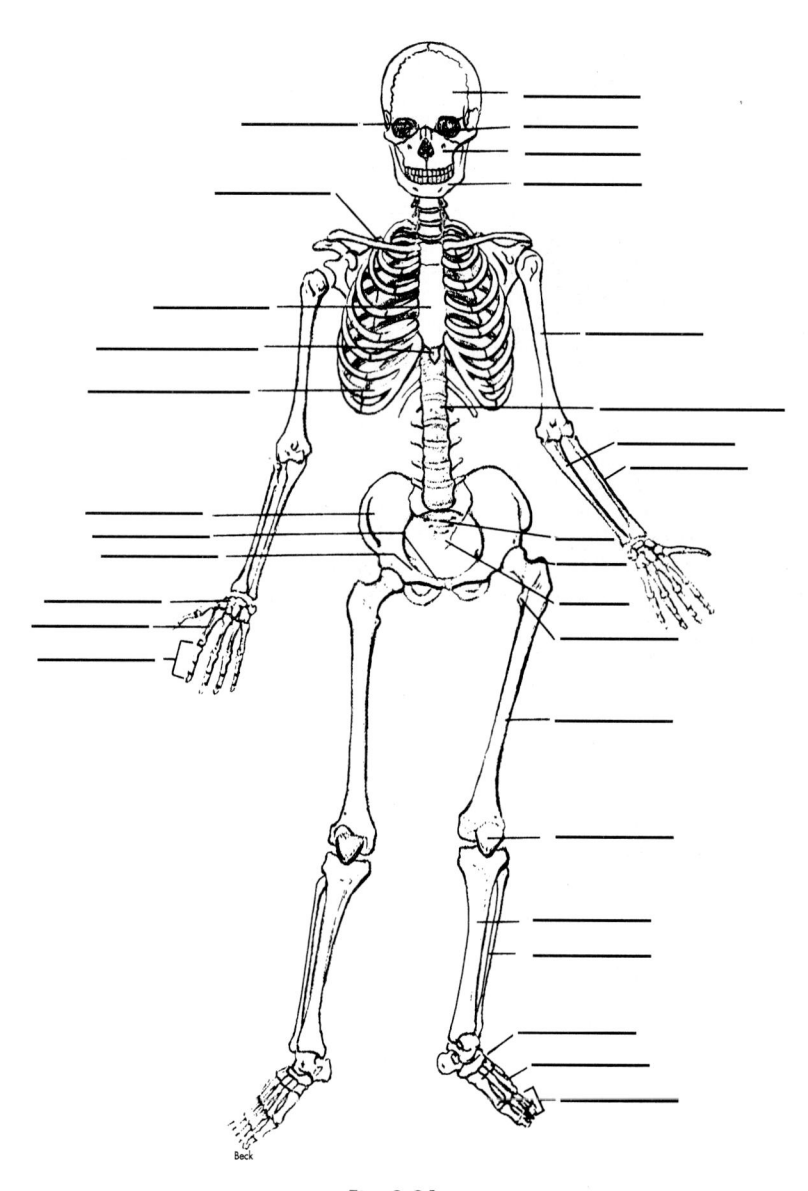

Fig. 3.2A

Label the skeletal system for Figure 3.2B that shows the posterior view of the skeleton.

aa. parietal bone
bb. occipital bone
cc. cervical vertebrae
dd. acromion process
ee. scapula
ff. thoracic vertebrae
gg. lumbar vertebrae
hh. ilium
ii. sacrum
jj. ischium
kk. humerus
ll. olecranon process of ulna
mm. radius
nn. ulna
oo. coccyx
pp. femur
qq. fibula
rr. tibia
ss. talus
tt. calcaneus

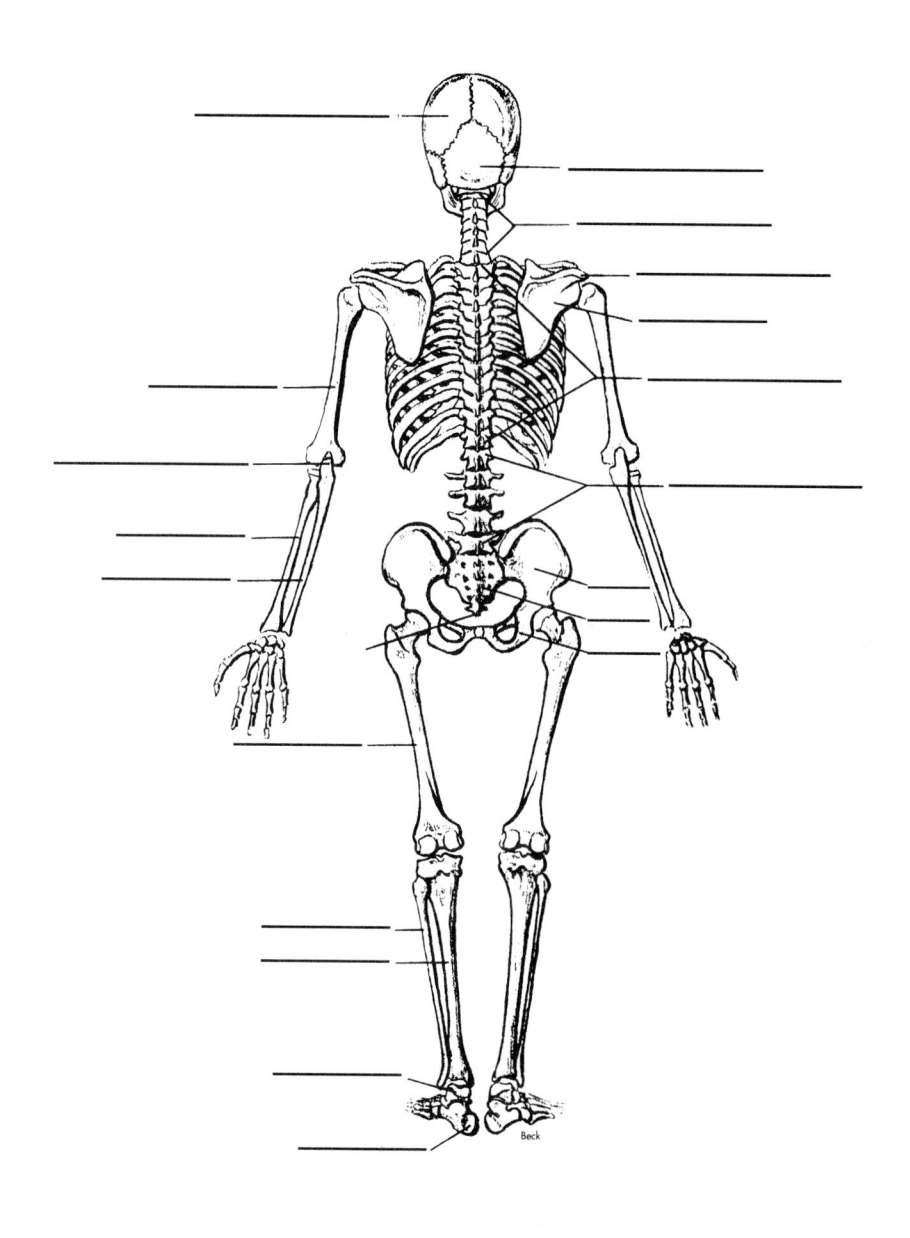

Fig. 3.2B

Label the types of diarthrotic joints for Figure 3.3.

A. ball and socket
B. saddle
C. condyloid
D. hinge
E. gliding
F. pivot

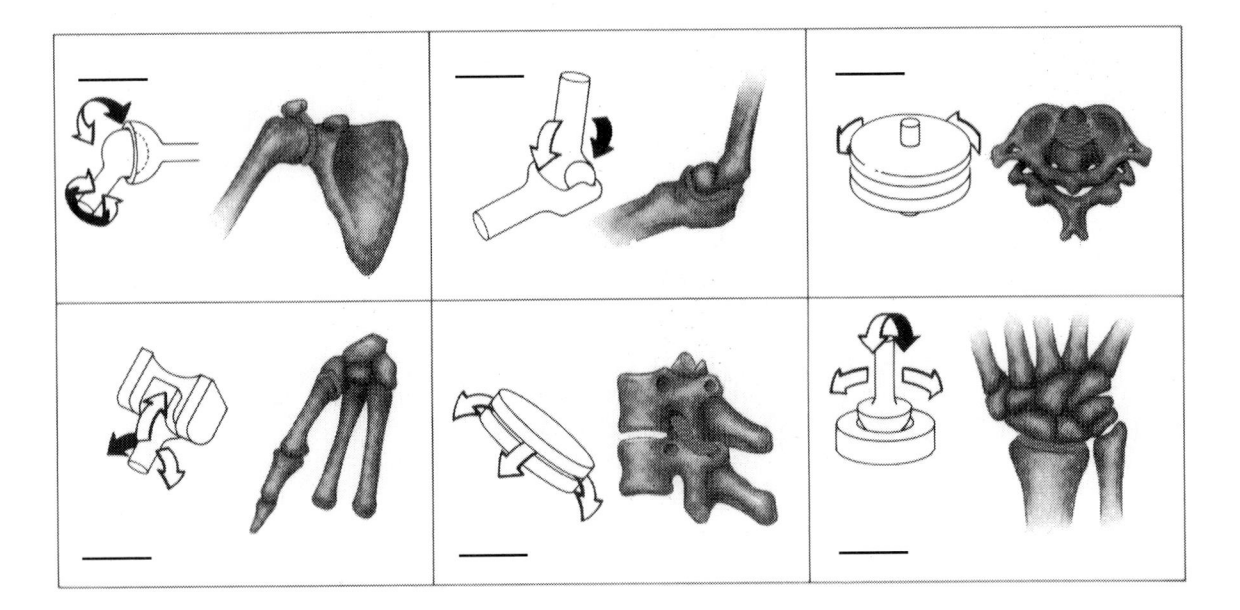

Fig. 3.3

Label the major superficial muscles for Figures 3.4 A and B. Some of these muscles show up on both sides of the body, but are listed here only once. Place the correct letter in both locations.

a. orbicularis oculi
b. orbicularis oris
c. brachialis
d. vastus medialis
e. frontalis
f. sternocleidomastoid
g. deltoid
h. pectoralis major
i. biceps brachii
j. rectus abdominis
k. rectus femoris
l. sartorius
m. peroneus longus

n. triceps brachii
o. extensor carpi ulnaris
p. flexor carpi ulnaris
q. trapezius
r. teres major
s. latissimus dorsi
t. gluteus medius
u. gluteus maximus
v. vastus lateralis
w. gastrocnemius
x. Achilles tendon
y. hamstrings

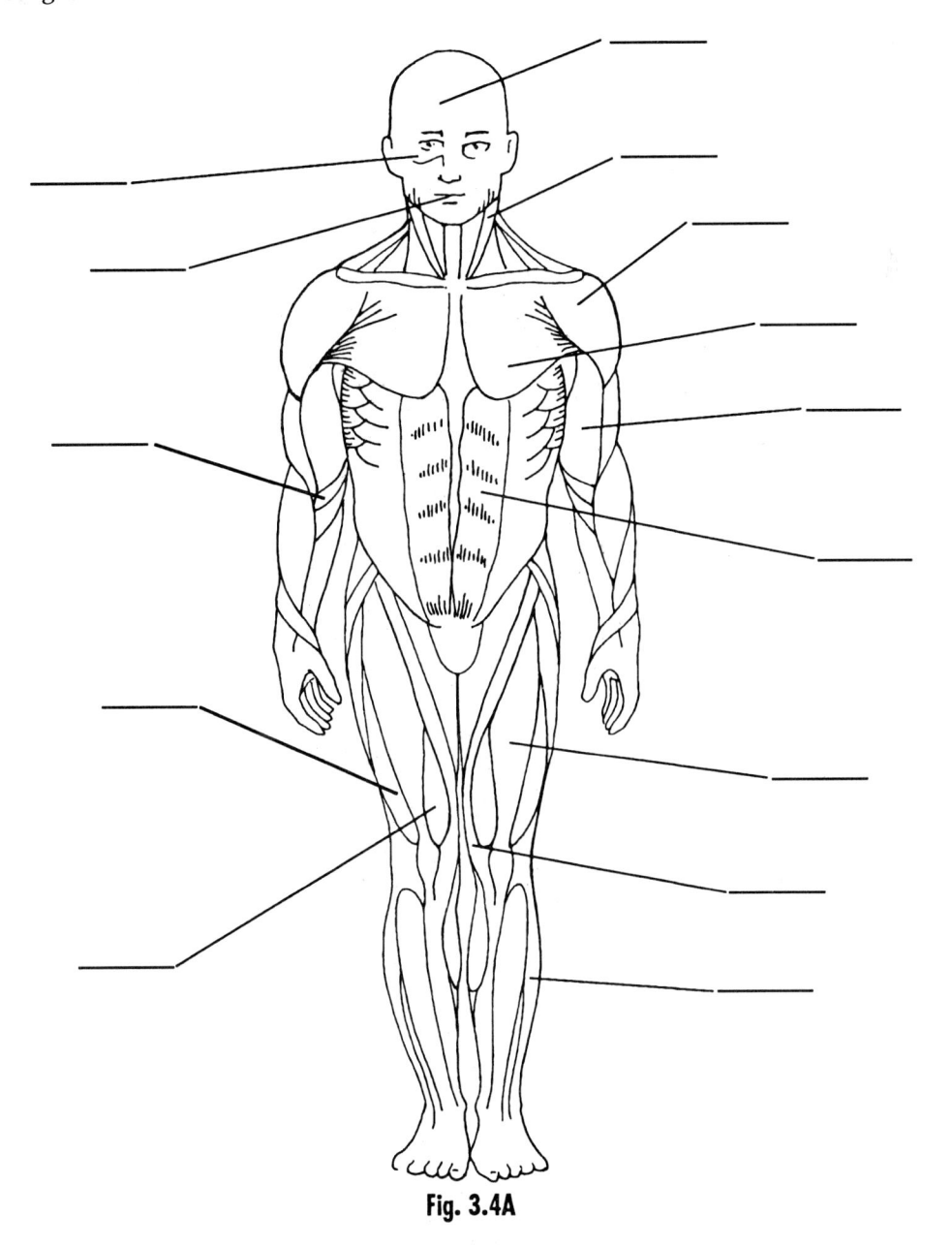

Fig. 3.4A

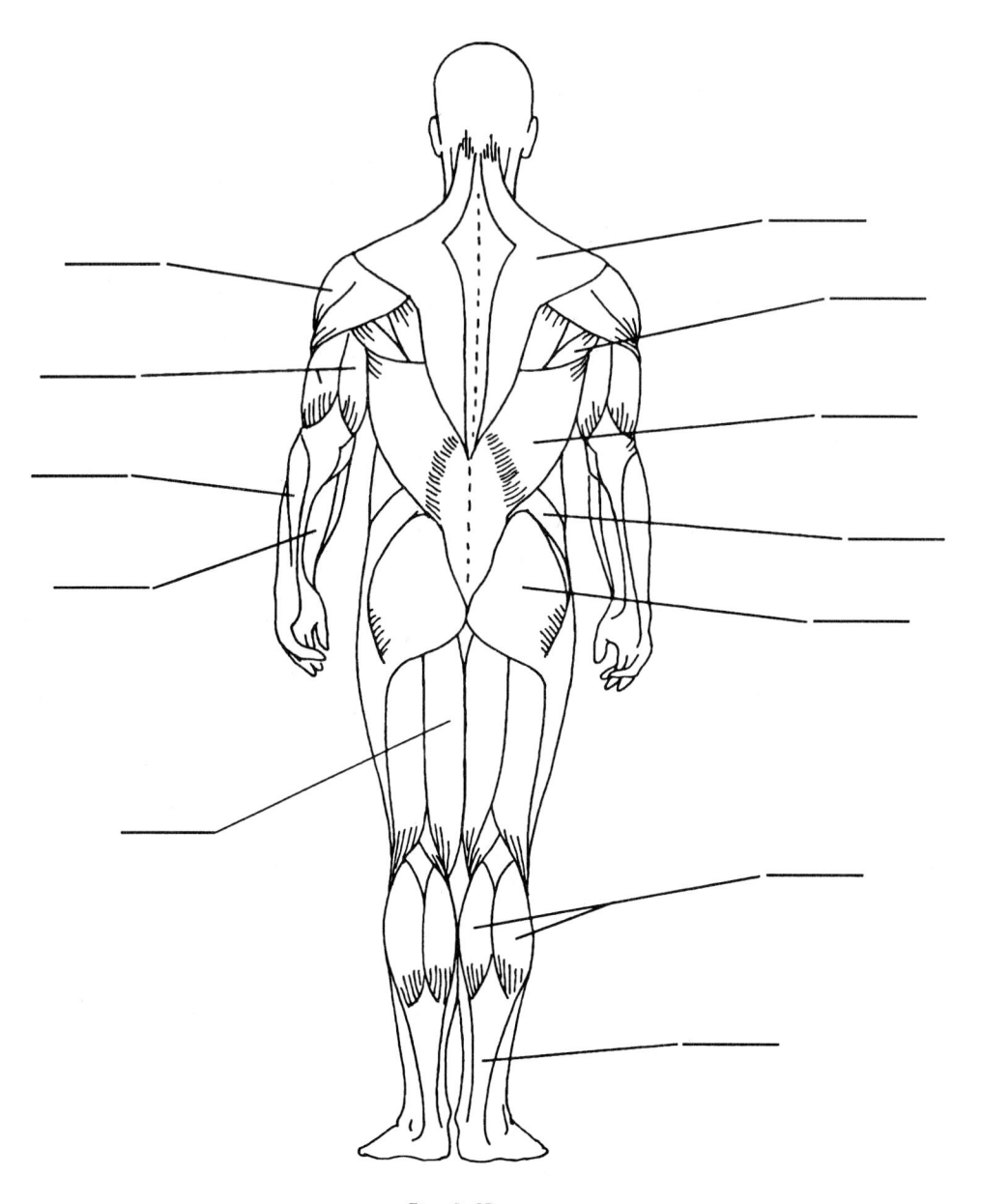

Fig. 3.4B

D. MATCHING

1. With each of the following word elements, match it to its proper meaning, then designate whether it is a prefix, root word, or suffix. Remember that some of the root words may not have a vowel at the end, since vowels are added only when combined with a suffix.

		MEANING	PREFIX, ROOT WORD, OR SUFFIX
1.	ab		
2.	ad		
3.	algia		
4.	arthro		
5.	chondr		
6.	circum		
7.	contra		
8.	cost		
9.	de		
10.	dia		
11.	dis		
12.	dys		
13.	epi		
14.	fibr		
15.	genesis		
16.	genic		
17.	gram		
18.	graph		
19.	graphy		
20.	hyper		
21.	inter		
22.	intra		
23.	intro		
24.	ism		
25.	itis		
26.	myo		
27.	myel		
28.	neuro		
29.	orth		
30.	osis		
31.	osteo		
32.	pathy		
33.	plegia		
34.	post		
35.	stasis		
36.	sterno		
37.	sub		
38.	supra		
39.	therm		
40.	thoraco		
41.	trans		
42.	vertebr		

a. toward
b. over, on, upon
c. producing, causing
d. a diagram, a recording instrument
e. excessive, too much, high
f. around
g. against, opposite
h. joint
i. record
j. a condition
k. away from
l. nerve
m. condition
n. making a recording
o. paralysis
p. maintenance, maintaining a constant level
q. across
r. spine, vertebrae
s. development, production, creation
t. pain
u. above, over
v. disease
w. chest
x. fiber, fibrous
y. cartilage
z. under
aa. heat
bb. rib
cc. bad, difficult, abnormal
dd. within
ee. down, from, away from, not
ff. across, through, apart
gg. inflammation
hh. spinal cord, bone marrow
ii. separation, away from
jj. between
kk. into, within
ll. straight, normal, correct
mm. bone
nn. after, behind
oo. sternum
pp. muscle

2. Match the lymph nodes and plexuses to their correct description.

1. parotid
2. occipital
3. superficial cervical
4. subclavicular
5. hypogastric
6. facial
7. deep cervical
8. axillary
9. mediastinal
10. cubital
11. para-aortic
12. deep inguinal
13. superficial inguinal
14. popliteal
15. mammary plexus
16. palmar plexus
17. plantar plexus

a. ____ deeply situated nodes in the groin.
b. ____ the nodes in the groin close to the surface.
c. ____ the nodes under the collarbone.
d. ____ the nodes draining the tissue in the face.
e. ____ lymphatic vessels in the sole (plantar) of the foot.
f. ____ lymphatic vessels in the palm (palmar) of the hands.
g. ____ the nodes around or in front of the ear.
h. ____ the nodes over the bone at the back of the head.
i. ____ the nodes in the area beneath the stomach.
j. ____ nodes around the aorta.
k. ____ deeply situated nodes in the neck.
l. ____ lymphatic vessels around the breasts.
m. ____ nodes in the armpit.
n. ____ nodes of the elbow.
o. ____ the nodes close to the surface of the neck.
p. ____ nodes in back of the knee.
q. ____ nodes in the mediastinal section of the thoracic cavity.

E. PROBLEM SOLVING EXERCISE

This week, six new clients come to your office. Each one of them has filled out a client history form ahead of time, providing you with the following information on the medical conditions that have been diagnosed and treated by their physicians. Take each of the italicized medical terms, and break it down into its word parts to define the various condition:

problems with *dermatitis* of the hands, *neuropathy* in the left leg, *hypothyroidism, dyspnea, hemangioma, polyarthritis, myocarditis, hydronephrosis*

F. PROFESSIONAL APPLICATION

A client brings in a research article about application of massage to a specific condition, but does not understand what is means. What steps would you take to explain the article to the client?

_____

_____

_____

_____

G. RESEARCH FOR FURTHER STUDY

List three resource books you could use for further study of medical terminology. Include title, publisher, and type of reference.

_____

_____

_____

ANSWERS

A. KEY TERMS

1. d
2. a
3. c
4. b
5. f
6. e

B. PUZZLE

1. anterior
2. valgus
3. plantar
4. recumbent
5. distal
6. medial
7. peripheral
8. volar
9. erect
10. supine
11. inferior
12. proximal
13. dorsal
14. lateral
15. superficial

C. LABELING

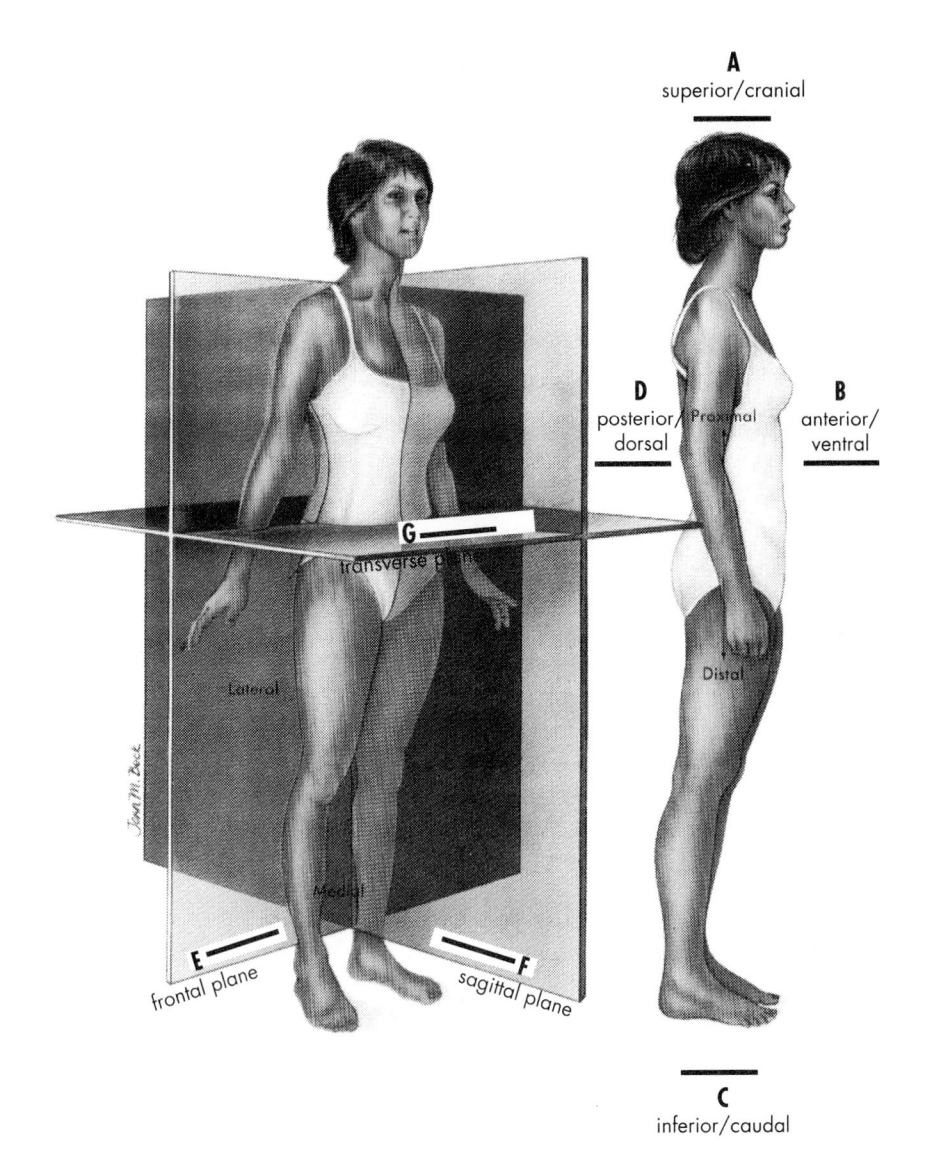

A superior/cranial

D posterior/dorsal

B anterior/ventral

Proximal

G transverse plane

Lateral

Distal

Medial

E frontal plane

F sagittal plane

C inferior/caudal

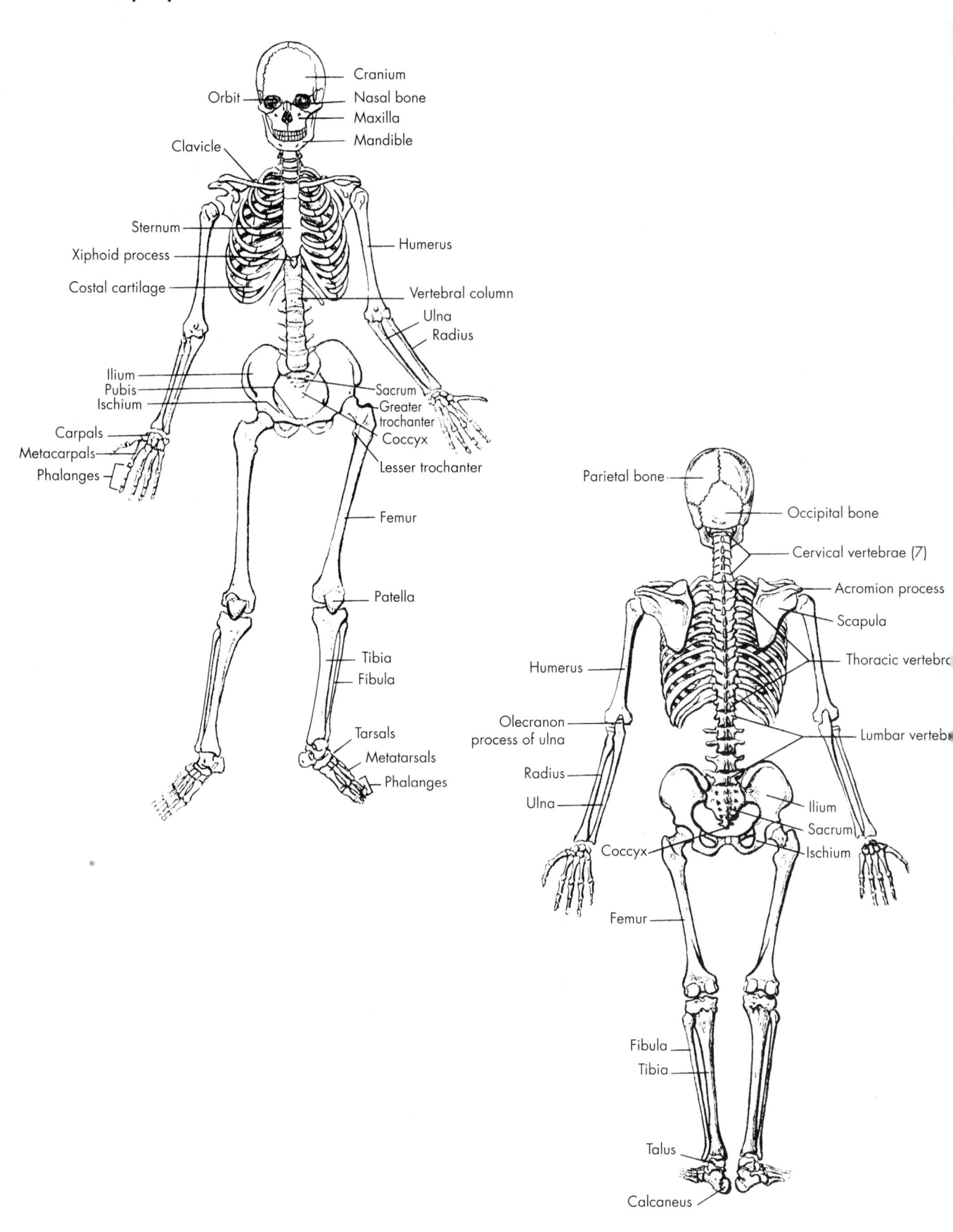

C. LABELING (cont.)

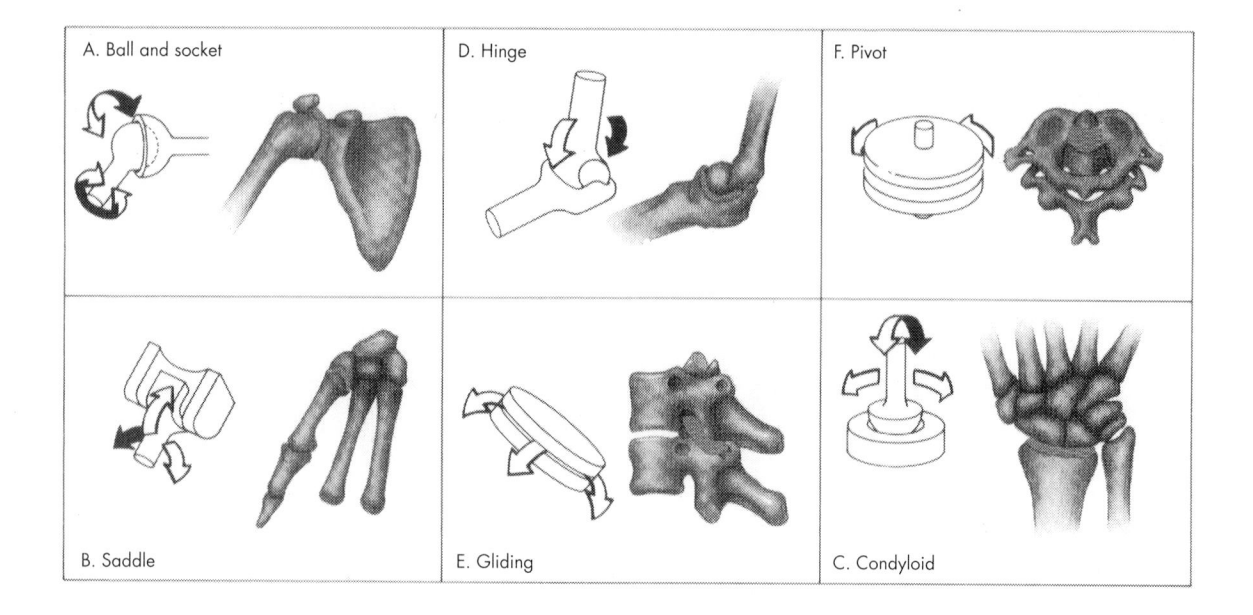

C. LABELING (cont.)

A. Ball and socket	D. Hinge	F. Pivot
B. Saddle	E. Gliding	C. Condyloid

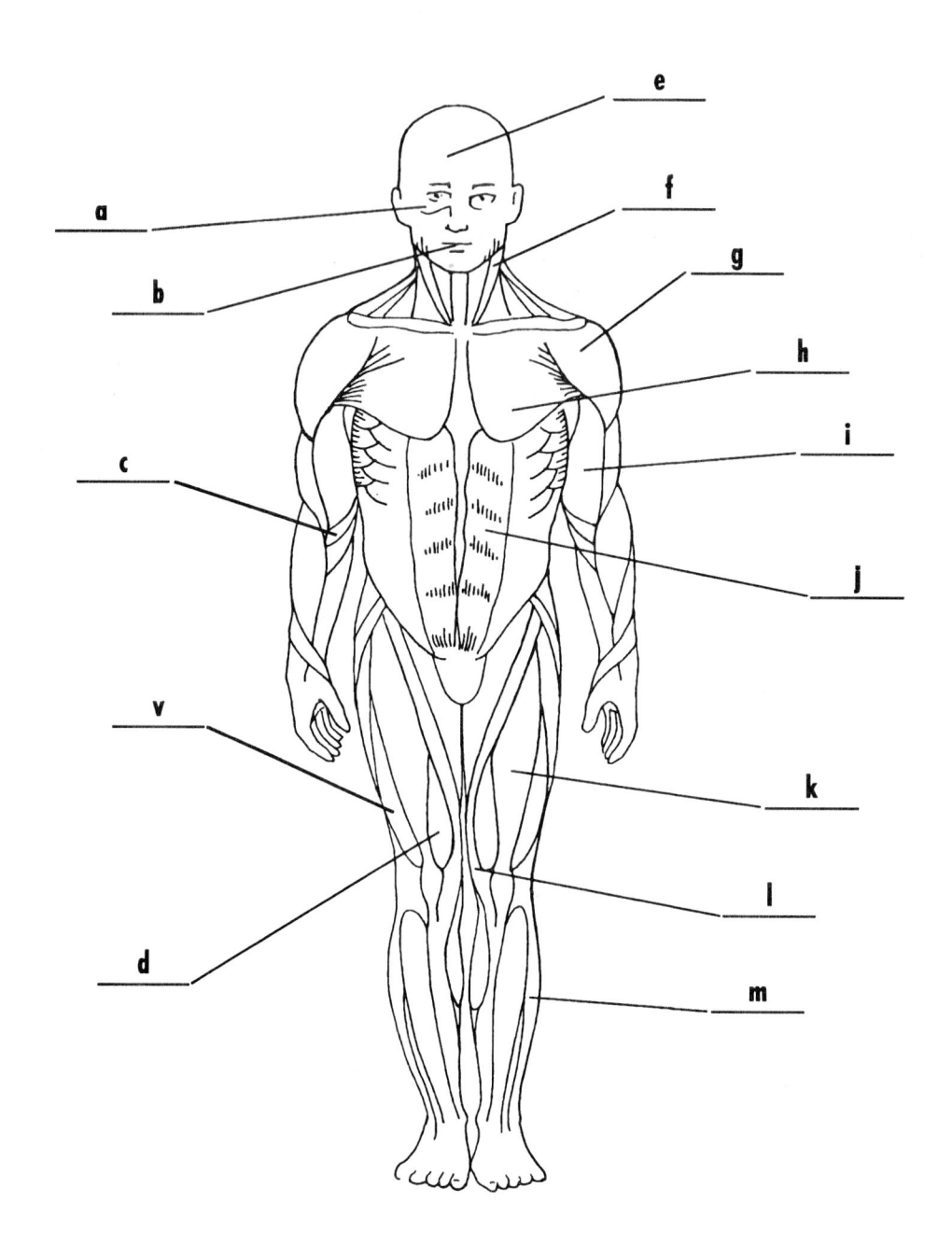

C. LABELING (cont.)

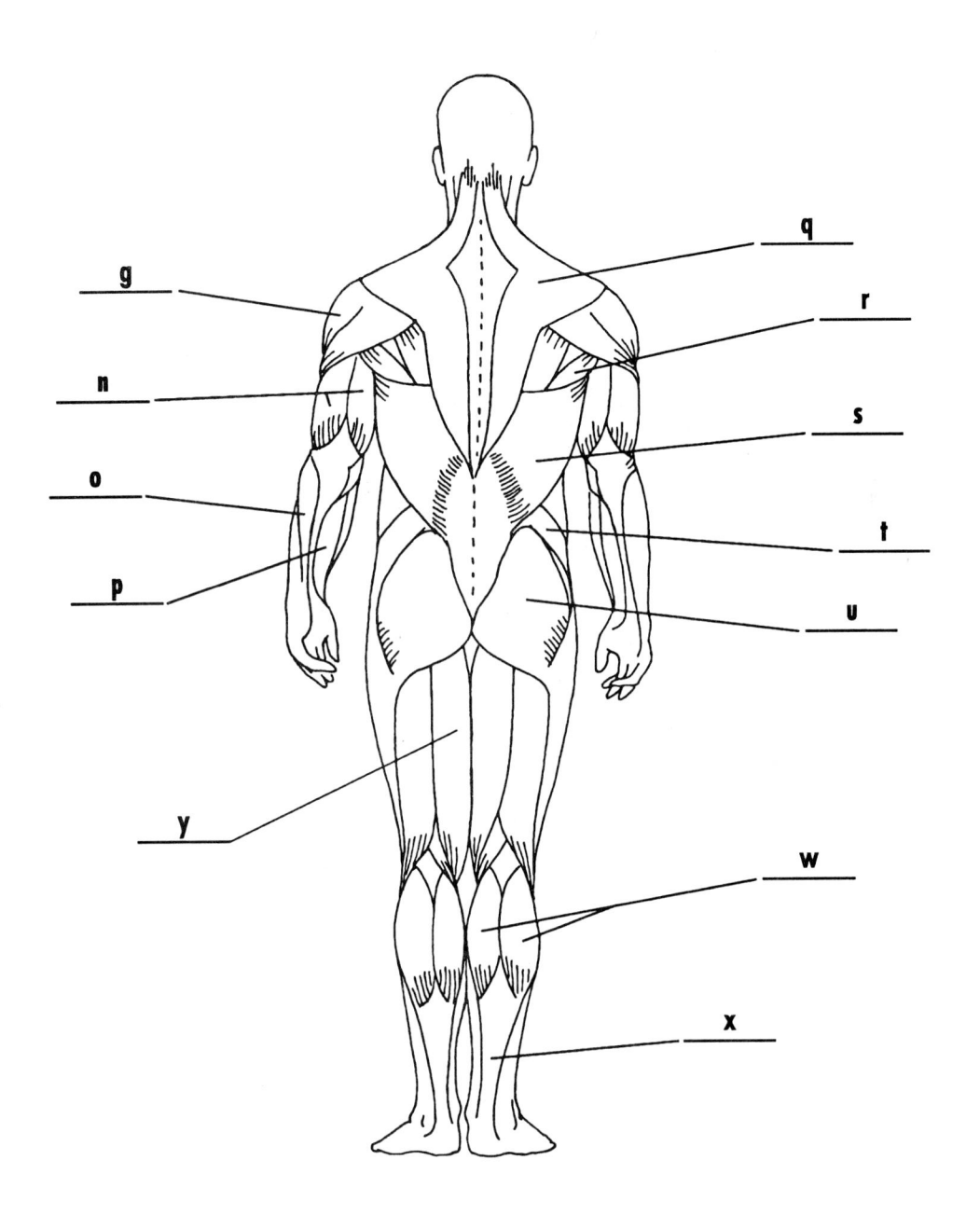

C. LABELING (cont.)

g
n
o
p
y
q
r
s
t
u
w
x

D. MATCHING

The first letter is the definition, the second letter indicates whether it is a prefix (p), root word (r), or suffix (s).

1. Word Elements:

1. k, p
2. a, p
3. t, s
4. h, r
5. y, r
6. f, p
7. g, p
8. bb, r
9. ee, p
10. ff, p
11. ii, p
12. cc, p
13. b, p
14. x, r
15. s, s
16. c, s
17. i, s
18. d, s
19. n, s
20. e, p
21. jj, p
22. dd, p
23. kk, p
24. j, s
25. gg, s
26. pp, r
27. hh, r
28. l, r
29. ll, r
30. m, s
31. mm, p
32. v, s
33. o, s
34. nn, p
35. p, s
36. oo, r
37. z, p
38. u, p
39. aa, r
40. w, r
41. q, p
42. r, r

2. Lymph Nodes and Plexuses:

1. g
2. h
3. o
4. c
5. i
6. d
7. k
8. m
9. q
10. n
11. j
12. a
13. b
14. p
15. l
16. f
17. e

E. PROBLEM SOLVING EXERCISE

Answers:

dermatitis: derma - skin   itis - inflammation
neuropathy: neuro - nerve   pathy - disease
hypothyroidism: hypo - less than normal   thyroid   ism - condition
dyspnea: dys - difficult   pnea - breathing
hemangioma: hemi - half   angi - vessel   oma - tumor (tumor made up of a mass of blood vessels)
polyarthritis: poly - many   arthr - joint   itis - inflammation
myocarditis: myo - muscle   card - heart   itis - inflammation
hydronephrosis: hydro - water   nephr - kidney   osis - condition

CHAPTER 4

Indications and Contraindications For Massage

A. KEY TERMS

Match the term to the best definition.

1. acute pain _____
2. arterial circulation _____
3. autonomic nervous system _____
4. cerebral spinal fluid _____
5. chronic diseases _____
6. chronic pain _____
7. connective tissue _____
8. contraindication _____
9. dermatome _____
10. dermatomal rule _____
11. disease _____
12. electrical-chemical _____
13. endangerment site _____
14. general contraindications _____
15. health _____
16. homeostasis _____
17. idiopathic _____
18. indication _____
19. inflammatory response _____
20. intractable pain _____

21. lymphatic drainage _____
22. metastasis _____
23. neuromuscular _____
24. pain _____
25. pain-spasm-pain cycle _____
26. pathology _____
27. phantom pain _____
28. piezoelectricity _____
29. referral _____
30. referred pain _____
31. regeneration _____
32. regional contraindications _____
33. replacement _____
34. respiration _____
35. risk factors _____
36. signs _____
37. somatic pain _____
38. state dependent memory _____
39. stress _____
40. symptoms _____

41. syndrome _____
42. venous circulation _____
43. visceral pain _____

a. When pain is referred, it is usually to a structure that developed from the same embryonic segment or dermatome as the structure in which the pain originates.
b. Cutaneous (skin) distribution of spinal nerve sensations.
c. Tumor cell migration by way of lymphatic or blood vessels.
d. An unpleasant sensory and emotional experience associated with actual or perceived tissue damage or described in terms of such damage.
e. The most abundant tissue of the body. Its functions include support, structure, space, stabilization, and scar formation.
f. A warning signal that activates the sympathetic nervous system, it can be a symptom of a disease condition, or a temporary aspect of medical treatment. It is usually temporary, of sudden onset, and easily localized.
g. The production of an electric current by application of pressure to certain crystals such as mica, quartz, Rochelle Salt, and some aspect of the connective tissue, most likely the collagen.
h. Dynamic equilibrium of the internal environment of the body through processes of feedback and regulation.
i. Diseases that develop slowly and last for a long time.
j. Pain arising from stimulation of receptors in the skin, or from stimulation of receptors in skeletal muscles, joints, tendons, and fascia.
k. Encoding and storage of a memory based on the autonomic nervous system and the resulting chemical balance of the body. The memory is only retrievable during a similar situation in the body.
l. Any substantial change in routine, or any activity which causes the body to have to adapt, including changes for the better, and changes for the worse.

m. A diffuse, poorly localized discomfort that persists or recurs for indefinite periods, usually for more than six months.
n. Regulates the energy using sympathetic "fight/flight/fear" response and the restorative parasympathetic "relaxation response." Sympathetic and parasympathetic systems work together to maintain homeostasis through a feedback loop system.
o. The subjective abnormalities felt only by the patient.
p. A collection of different signs and symptoms, usually with a common cause, that present a clear picture of a pathological condition.
q. The return of deoxygenated blood to the heart by way of the veins.
r. Pain that results from stimulation of receptors in the internal organs.
s. An abnormality in a body function that threatens well-being.
t. A liquid that nourishes and protects the brain and nerves.
u. Movement of oxygenated blood under pressure from the heart to the body through the arteries.
v. Healing process where the new cells are formed from connective tissue. The cells are different from those that they replace, resulting in a scar.
w. Healing process where the new cells are similar to those that they replace.
x. Method to send a client to a health care professional for specific diagnosis and treatment of a disease.
y. The interaction between the control and response of the muscles to nerve signals.
z. A therapeutic application that promotes health or assists in a healing process.
aa. Any condition that renders a particular treatment improper or undesirable.
bb. A normal mechanism that usually speeds recovery from an infection or injury characterized by pain, heat, redness, and swelling.
cc. Physiologic functions of the body that rely on or produce body energy in some form. Often called chi, prana, meridian energy, etc.

dd. Physical, mental, and social well-being – not merely the absence of disease.

ee. The study of disease.

ff. A kind of pain frequently experienced by patients who have had a limb amputated.

gg. The steady contraction of muscles causing them to become ischemic, which stimulates the pain receptors in the muscles. The pain, in turn, initiates more spasms, setting up a vicious circle.

hh. A specific type of massage that enhances lymphatic flow.

ii. Chronic pain that persists even when treatment is provided, or it exists without demonstrable disease.

jj. Diseases with undetermined causes.

kk. Area of the body where nerves and blood vessels surface close to the skin and are not well protected by muscle or connective tissue. Deep sustained pressure into these areas could damage these vessels and nerves.

ll. Those findings that require a physician's evaluation to rule out serious underlying conditions before any massage is indicated.

mm. Contraindications that relate to a specific area of the body.

nn. Movement of oxygen in the body during breathing.

oo. Predisposing conditions that may make the development of a disease more likely to occur.

pp. Objective abnormalities that can be seen or measured by someone other than the client.

qq. Pain felt in an area different than the source of the pain.

B. FILL IN THE BLANKS

The techniques of therapeutic massage and other types and styles of bodywork are merely _____ of the fundamental application of manual manipulations. The effectiveness of the techniques is a result of basic _____ effects.

It is unusual to encounter soft tissue (muscle and connective tissue) dysfunction without _____ hyperactivity. The result of proprioceptive hyperactivity is tense or spastic muscles, accompanied by hypoactivity of _____ groups of muscles. When working with the _____ mechanism, the basic premise is to substitute a different neurological signal stimulation through massage, to reset muscle resting length through lengthening and stretching muscles and connective tissue, and to provide re-education of the muscles involved. The basic premise when working with _____ is to provide space and mobile stability, as opposed to the dysfunctional joint or soft tissue area which may be "stuck" and restricted or hypermobile. This is accomplished through _____, sustained pulling and _____ of the connective tissue, and frictioning methods.

Massage and other forms of bodywork mimic and assist the _____ action of the muscle and respiratory pump.

An increase in _____ flow is beneficial in any situation in which an increase in oxygenated blood is desirable. Such situations include sluggish circulation or an increased demand such as with an athlete.

Venous return flow is dependent on _____ of the muscles against the veins. Passive and active _____ movement also encourages the muscles to contract against the deeper vessels, assisting venous blood flow. The procedures for _____ are the same as those for venous return. Because lymph vessels are open-ended into all tissue space the surface work is performed over the _____ body instead of being focused only over the major veins. Beneficial effects of massage include _____ breathing. Techniques of cranial-sacral therapy specifically affect _____ circulation. The basic premise when working with circulation enhancement is to provide for a sufficient, even, and _____ circulatory flow.

Examples of methods used for _____ are ice, heat, counter-irritation, topical ointments, acupressure, acupuncture, rocking, music, and repetitive massage methods. Because of the generalized effect on the ANS and associated functions, massage can produce changes in mood and excitement levels, and can induce the _____. The basic premise of a massage focused on the ANS is to provide for a balanced mind/body state that allows for efficient _____.

Physiologically, acupuncture points and meridians can be correlated directly to the _____ and motor nerve points; chakras are located over nerve plexuses; and connective tissue techniques produce a measurable _____ current via the piezoelectric properties of the connective tissue. The basic premise when working with the energy systems of the body is to provide an unobstructed _____ of energy. Whatever the massage or bodywork system used, the beneficial effects of therapeutic massage are elicited from the client's _____ as it adjusts to the external _____ information supplied by massage and responds to the compressive forces of massage.

C. PUZZLE

Complete the puzzle by filling in the spaces with the following words.

acute
arterial circulation
chronic pain
endangerment site
idiopathic
inflamed
lymphatic
malignant
metastasis
neoplasm
neuromuscular
pain
referral
signs
stress

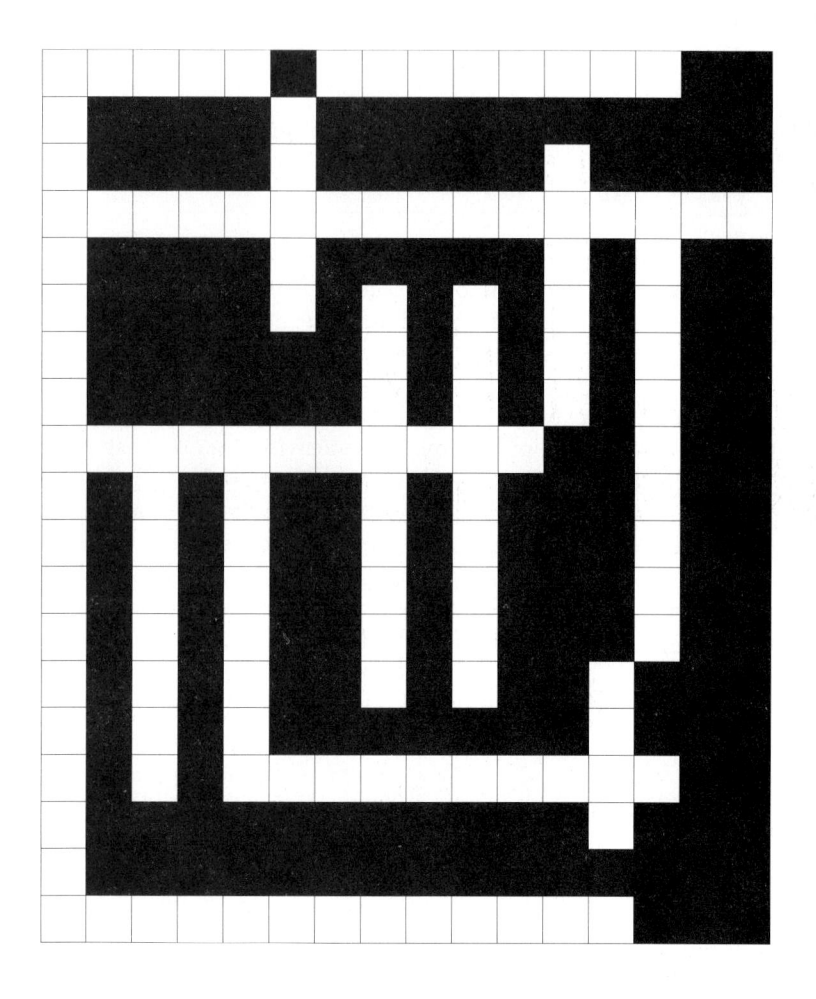

D. LABELING

Label the areas of referred pain for Figure 4.1.

A. Urinary bladder
B. Colon
C. Appendix
D. Heart
E. Lung and diaphragm
F. Liver and gallbladder
G. Ovary
H. Pancreas
I. Small intestine
J. Kidney
K. Stomach

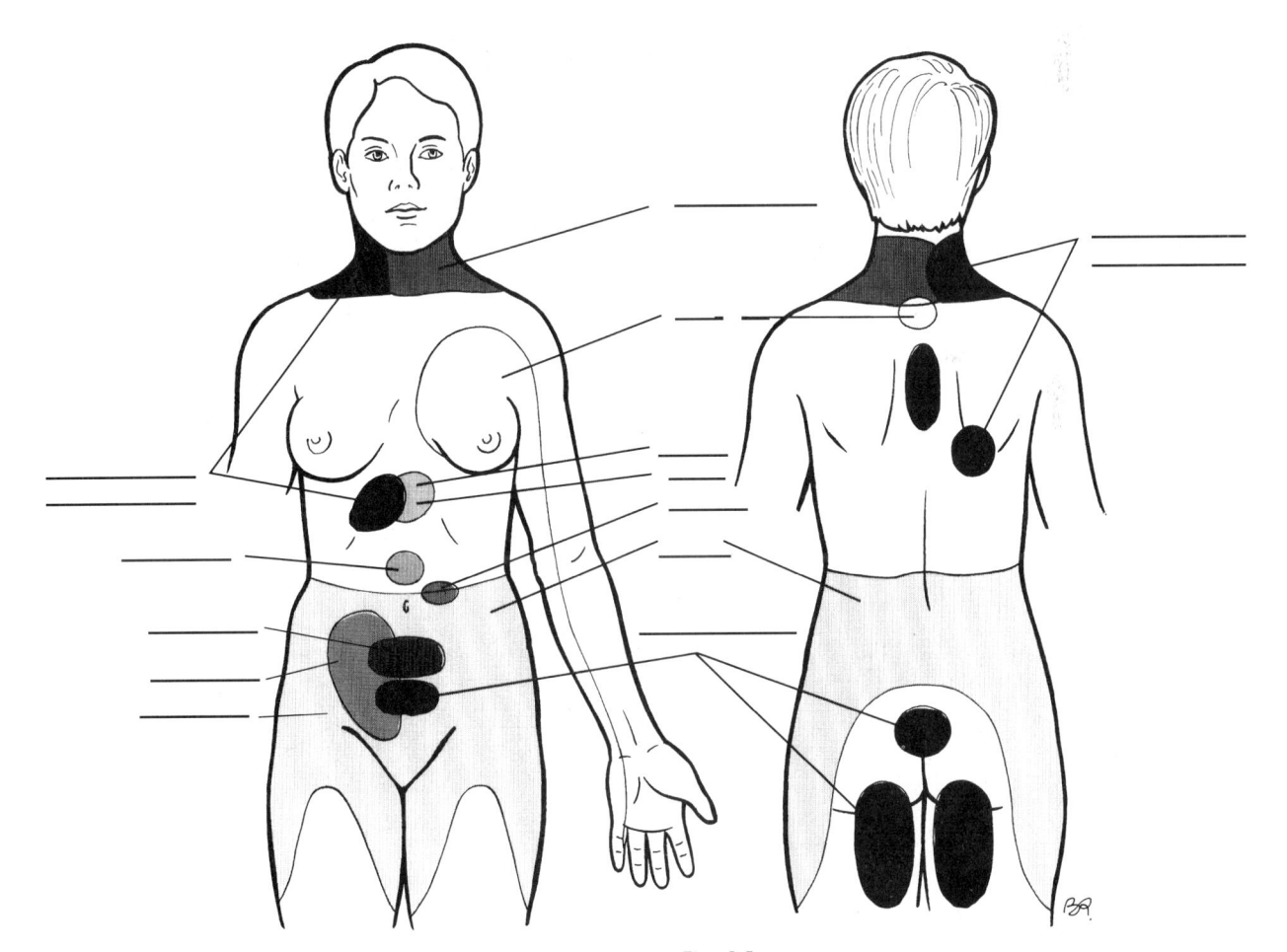

Fig. 4.1

Indications and Contraindications For Massage

Label the endangerment sites for Figure 4.2.

A. Anterior triangle of neck
B. Posterior triangle of neck
C. Axillary area
D. Ulnar nerve
E. Radial nerve
F. Vagus nerve, nerves and vessels to thyroid gland
G. Abdominal and descending aorta
H. Kidney
I. Sciatic nerve
J. Inguinal triangle
K. Tibial nerve, popliteal artery and nerve

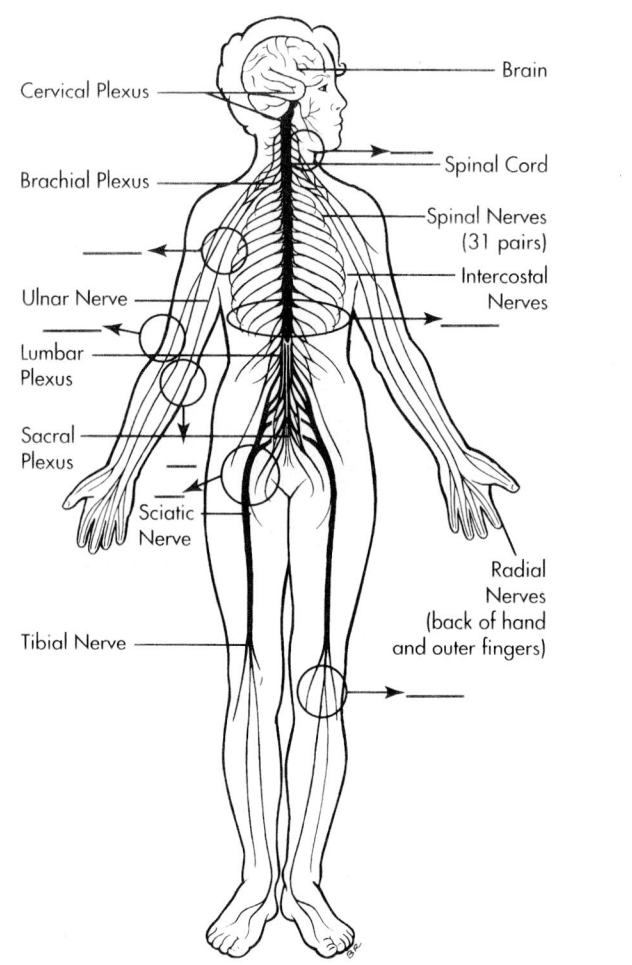

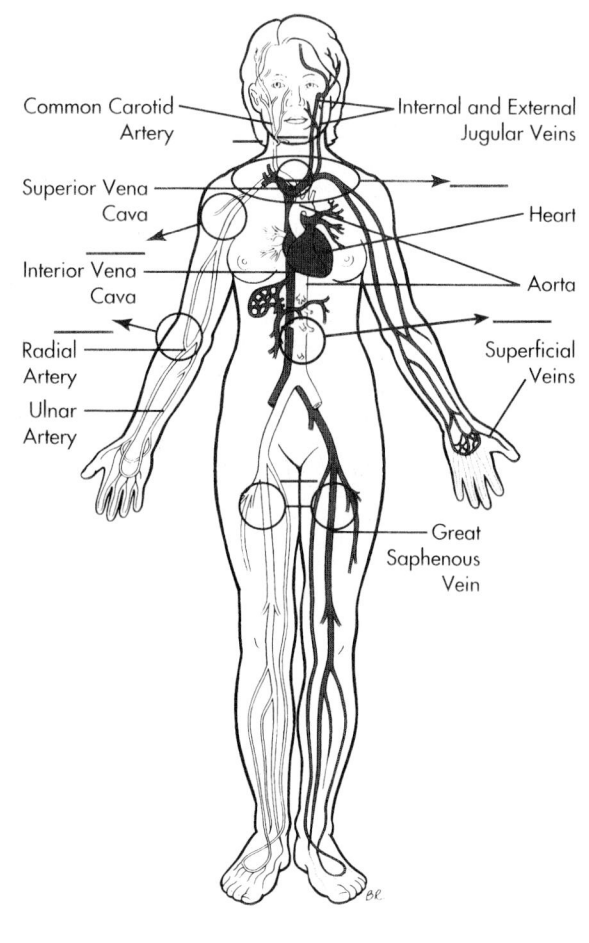

Fig. 4.2

E. MATCHING

Match the correct words with the primary responses:

1. Heat and Redness
2. Swelling and Pain

   a. histamine, prostaglandins, and kinins are released _____
   b. increased permeability of vessel walls _____
   c. enlargement of lymph nodes _____
   d. dilation of blood vessels _____
   e. edema pressure triggers pain receptors _____
   f. irritant diluted through excess fluid _____
   g. white blood cells destroy bacteria _____
   h. increase in blood volume _____

F. ADDITIONAL ACTIVITIES

Risk Factors

1. List all the risk factors for developing disease, and write down separate columns for your personal risk factors, and the risk factors of two friends.

_____
_____
_____
_____
_____
_____

2. When interviewing a client or doing a massage, how would you find out if that person has any possible warning signs for cancer? A list of the signs is found below; state how or when you would find out the information if the client did not reveal it.

The warning signs of cancer:

Sores that do not heal

Unusual bleeding

A change in a wart or mole

A lump or thickening in any tissue

Persistent hoarseness or cough

Chronic indigestion

A change in bowel or bladder function

Example:

Sores that do not heal:
Noticed during proper draping techniques – skin on body has open wounds.

_____
_____
_____
_____
_____
_____
_____

G. PROBLEM SOLVING EXERCISE

You just ran into a friend you have not seen in five years. That friend is now a college professor, teaching anatomy and physiology. When you mention you are studying massage, the friend says, " It sounds interesting, but I don't think I'd ever need one." Take five minutes to list all the reasons you think your friend may need a massage.

_____
_____
_____
_____
_____
_____
_____

ANSWERS

A. KEY TERMS

1. f
2. u
3. n
4. t
5. i
6. m
7. e
8. aa
9. b
10. a
11. s
12. cc
13. kk
14. ll
15. dd
16. h
17. jj
18. z
19. bb
20. ii
21. hh
22. c
23. y
24. d
25. gg
26. ee
27. ff
28. g
29. x
30. qq
31. w
32. mm
33. v
34. nn
35. oo
36. pp
37. j
38. k
39. l
40. o
41. p
42. q
43. r

B. FILL IN THE BLANKS

variations
physiologic

proprioceptive
opposing
neuromuscular
connective tissue
mechanical compression
elongation

pumping

arterial

contraction
joint
lymphatic drain
entire
enhanced
cerebral spinal fluid
unobstructed

hyper-stimulation analgesia
relaxation response
self-regulation

nerve tracts
electrical
flow
physiology
sensory

C. PUZZLE

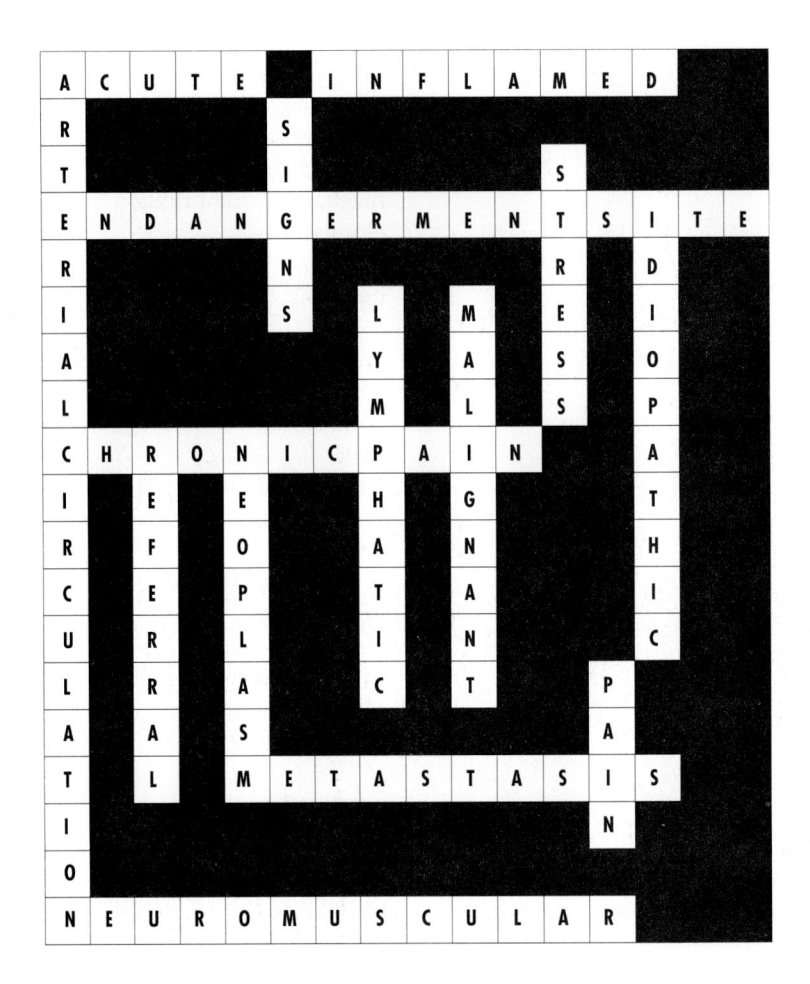

```
A C U T E . I N F L A M E D
R . . S . . . . . . .
T . . I . . . S . . .
E N D A N G E R M E N T S I T E
R . . N . . . R . D . .
I . . S . L . M . R . I .
A . . . . Y . A . E . O .
L . . . . M . L . S . P .
C H R O N I C P A I N . A .
I . E . E . H . G . . T .
R . F . O . A . N . . H .
C . E . P . T . A . . I .
U . R . L . I . N . . C .
L . R . A . C . T . P .
A . A . S . . . . . A .
T . L . M E T A S T A S I S
I . . . . . . . . . N .
O . . . . . . . . . . .
N E U R O M U S C U L A R
```

D. LABELING

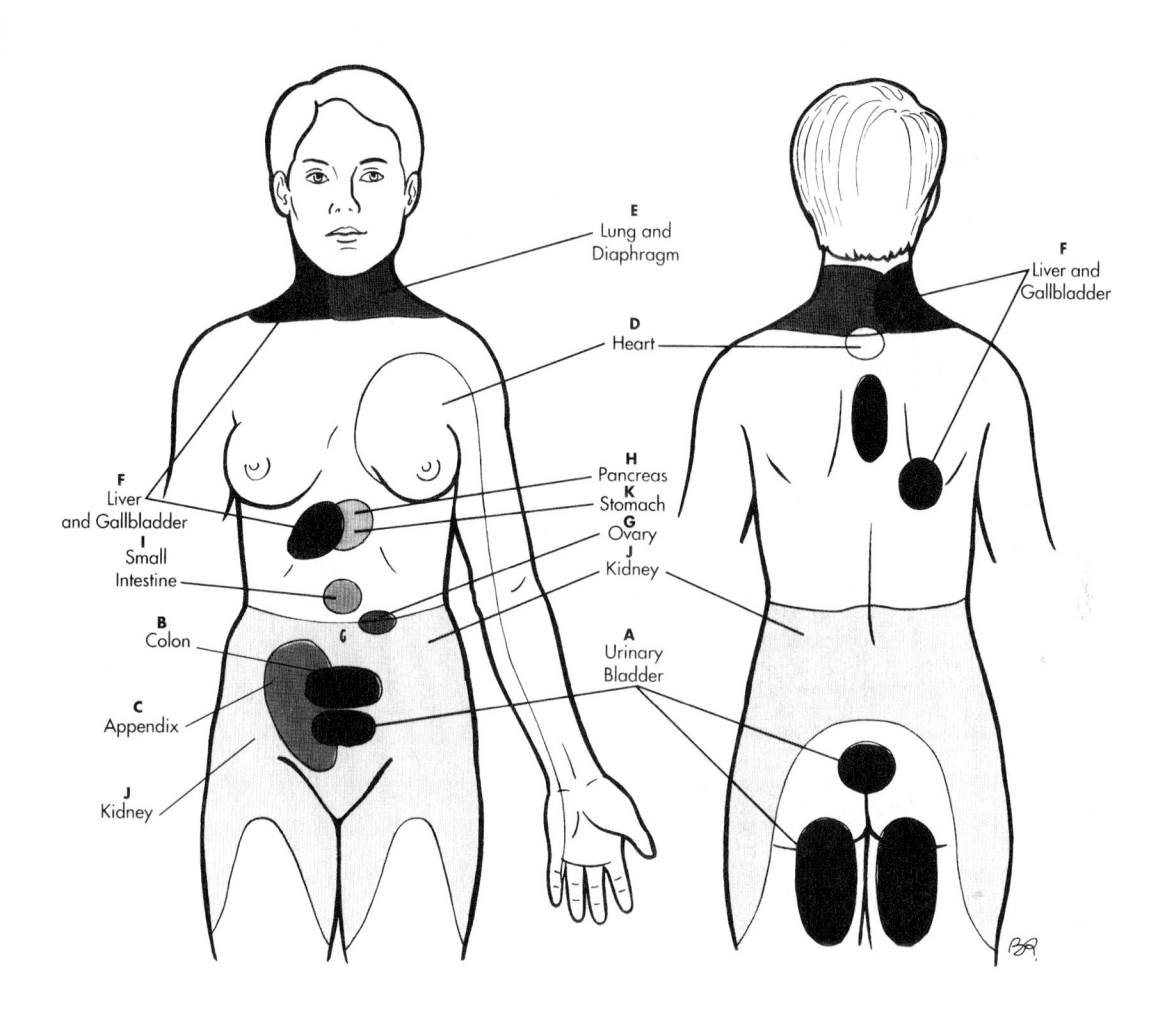

E — Lung and Diaphragm
D — Heart
F — Liver and Gallbladder
H — Pancreas
K — Stomach
G — Ovary
J — Kidney
I — Small Intestine
B — Colon
C — Appendix
J — Kidney
A — Urinary Bladder
F — Liver and Gallbladder

Indications and Contraindications For Massage

D. LABELING (cont.)

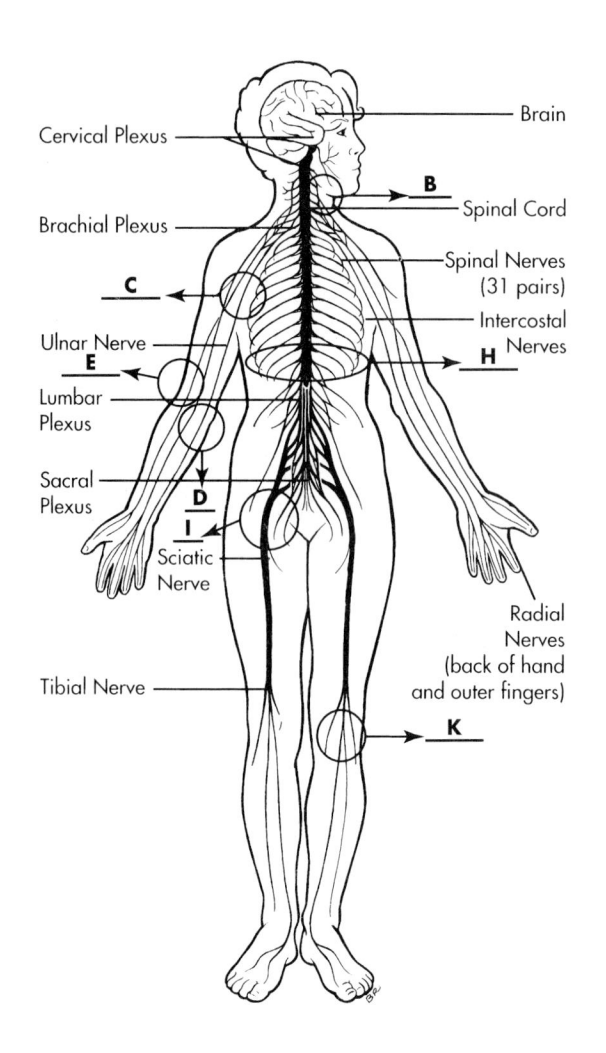

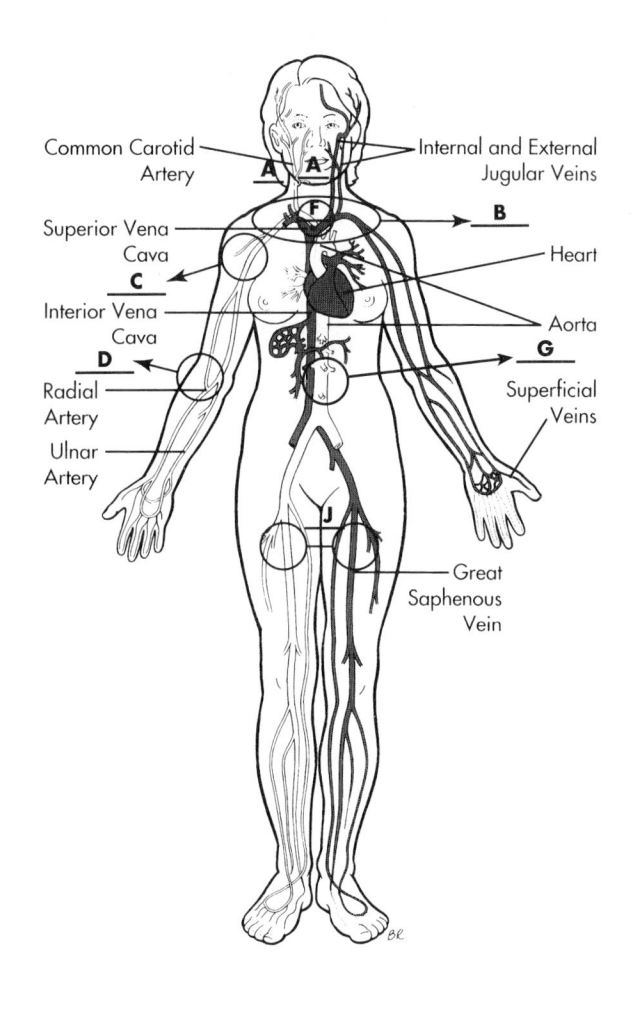

E. MATCHING

Match the correct words with the primary responses:

1. a, d, h
2. b, c, e, f, g

CHAPTER 5

Hygiene, Sanitation, and Safety

A. KEY TERMS

Match the term to the best definition.

1. AIDS _____
2. asepsis _____
3. Centers for Disease Control _____
4. communicable disease _____
5. contamination _____
6. dermatosis _____
7. dermatitis _____
8. disinfection _____
9. first aid _____
10. hazard _____
11. hemorrhage _____
12. host _____
13. hygiene _____
14. HIV _____
15. infection _____
16. microorganism _____
17. pathogen _____
18. sanitation _____
19. shock _____
20. sterilization _____
21. transmission _____
22. universal precautions _____

a. The absence of pathogens.
b. The excessive loss of blood from a blood vessel.
c. The human immunodeficiency virus.
d. The formulation and application of measures to promote and establish conditions favorable to health, in particular public health.
e. The process by which an object or area becomes unclean.
f. Procedures developed by the CDC to prevent the spread of contagious disease.
g. A disease caused by pathogens that are easily spread, a contagious disease.
h. Skin inflammation.

i. A condition that results when there is an inadequate blood supply to the organs and tissues of the body.
j. The process by which all microorganisms are destroyed.
k. A disease state that results from the invasion and growth of microorganisms in the body.
l. The person, animal, or environment in which microorganisms live and grow.
m. Acquired immune deficiency syndrome.
n. A small living plant or animal that cannot be seen without the aid of a microscope.
o. A microorganism that is harmful and capable of causing an infection. A virus, bacteria, fungus, protozoa, or pathogenic animal.
p. Emergency care given to an ill or injured person before medical help arrives.
q. Spread or transfer of pathogen.
r. The process by which pathogens are destroyed.
s. A division of the U.S. Public Health Service that investigates and controls various diseases, especially those that have epidemic potential.
t. Any skin condition.
u. Anything that poses a safety threat.
v. Practices and conditions for the promotion of health and the prevention of disease.

B. FILL IN THE BLANKS

One of the best ways to control disease is to stay _____. Smoking is considered one of the _____ causes of disease. Because the massage therapist works physically close to the client, any smoke _____ from the therapist are reason for concern. Because they affect thinking, feeling, behavior, and functioning, the therapist must never be under the influence of _____ or drugs when working with a client.

The massage therapist must pay careful attention to personal _____. The massage therapist should not wear perfume, aftershave, or perfumed hair products. Many clients are _____ to these odors. Hair must not fall onto the _____ of the therapist or drag on the client. Nails should be _____ and well manicured. Any hangnails, breaks, or cracks in the skin of the hands must be kept clean and _____ during a massage. Massage_____ should be loose and made of a cotton or cotton blend. Clothing should be_____ in a disinfectant, usually a bleach. If the client or the therapist is ill, and there is any concern that the condition is_____, the massage therapist should refer or reschedule the client until the condition changes.

_____ methods promote conditions that are conducive to health. That means that pathogenic organisms must be eliminated or controlled. _____ invade cells and insert their own genetic code into the host cell's genetic code. _____ are primitive cells without nuclei. They produce disease by secreting toxic substances that damage human tissues, by becoming parasites inside human cells, or by forming colonies in the body that disrupt normal human function. _____ are a group of simple parasitic organisms similar to plants but without chlorophyll (green pigment). _____ are small, single-celled fungi, and _____ are large, multi-cellular fungi. Fungal or mycotic infections often resist treatment, so they can become quite serious. _____ are one-celled organisms larger than bacteria that can infest human fluids and cause disease by parasitizing (living off) or directly destroying cells. Pathogenic animals, sometimes called metazoa, are large, multi-cellular organisms. Most are _____ that feed off human tissue or cause other disease processes.

The key to preventing many diseases caused by pathogenic organisms is to _____ organisms from entering the human body. Proper _____ is the single most effective deterrent to the spread of disease. Universal precautions issued by the CDC in 1987, _____ the spread of both bacterial and viral infections. We need to use universal precautions to _____ the client from viruses and bacteria. Any person touching a spill of blood or other body substance, such as vomit, urine, or feces, should wear single-use disposable _____. To clean up spills of body fluids, a 10% _____ solution should be used. If a contaminated substance comes into contact with human skin, the skin should be washed off immediately with _____ and water and an antiviral agent such as 10% bleach solution. A bleach and water solution should be prepared daily. Massage professionals should update their information on recommended sanitary practices at least every six months.

The massage therapist's facility must be kept _____ free.

The following safety rules are guidelines for providing a hazard-free massage environment. _____ and young children should not be left _____. Parents or guardians should always be present during massage for _____. Women in the last trimester of a _____ should not be left in the massage room alone and may need _____ getting on and off the massage table. The _____ may be less steady on their feet and should not be left in the massage room unattended. Anyone who is mobility impaired, including the visually-impaired, may need assistance getting on and off the massage table. Those with _____ should be asked what assistance they need, and their instructions followed carefully.

Preventing falls is very important. To prevent falls: Provide good _____. Never perform a massage in a dark room. Avoid loose _____ as they may slip or tangle in the feet. Avoid slippery tile floors. Keep floors and walkways _____. Keep cords out of _____ areas. Regularly check all massage _____ to make sure that it is in good repair. Make sure that all outside _____ are free from clutter and hazards from ice and rain.

Fire prevention is essential. To prevent fire: Provide for a _____ environment. Where smoking is allowed, make sure proper ashtrays are used. Empty ash trays only into a _____ that is partially filled with sand or water. Regularly check all _____ and equipment to make sure that they are in good condition. Do not plug more than _____ plugs into an electrical outlet. Never use candles, incense, or any other _____ flame. Make sure the massage area is equipped with a _____ detector and fire extinguisher. Check them regularly to make sure they are functional. If an accident does occur, the information about the accident must be written down.

C. PUZZLE

Complete the crossword puzzle by supplying answers to the following clues.

ACROSS:
2. A substance that destroy pathogens
5. A person or environment in which microorganisms live
7. Practices that promote health and prevent disease
8. A condition that will not maintain pathogens
10. Hazard free
12. Parasitic organisms without chlorophyll
13. Organism that invades living cells in order to use their genetic material
14. Conditions conducive to health

DOWN:
1. A microorganism capable of causing an infection
2. Skin inflammation
3. Universal guidelines which prevent the spread of bacteria and viruses
4. Actions that promote health and decrease the risk of illness or hazard
6. Waiting for or using the right conditions
9. Referring to equipment, activities, or techniques used in a clinic setting
11. A threat to safety

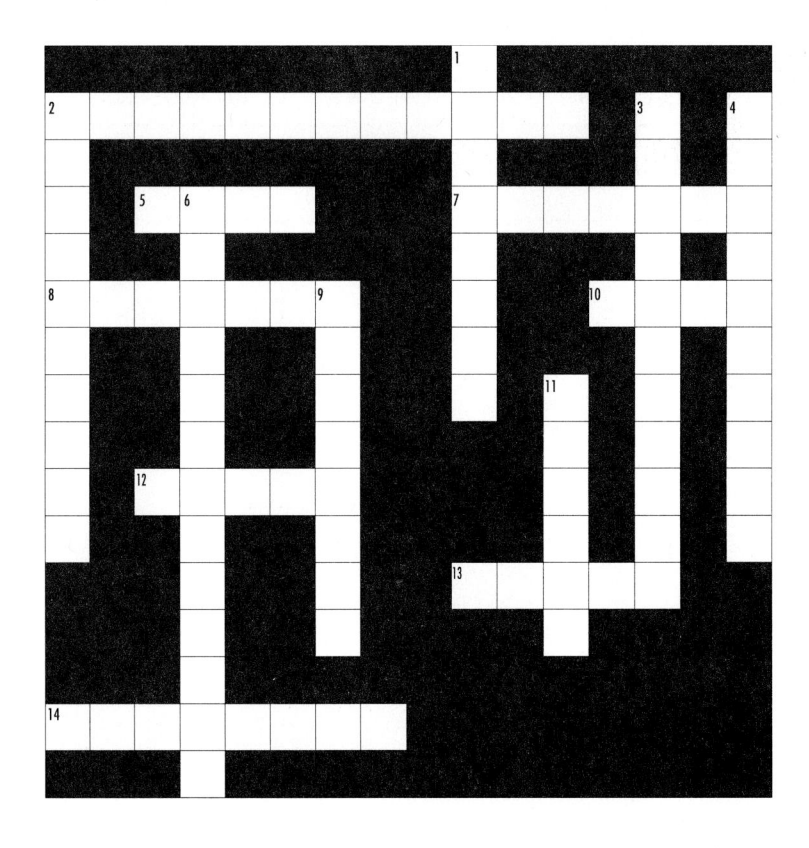

D. MATCHING

Match the ways that pathogens can be spread or controlled with the proper description.

1. _____ Pressurized steam bath, extreme temperature, or radiation.
2. _____ Chemicals such as iodine, chlorine, alcohol, and soaps.
3. _____ Quarantine of affected patients; protective apparel worn while giving treatments.
4. _____ Pathogens are found in the environment in food, water, soil, and on assorted surfaces.
5. _____ Disease is not caused until the pathogens have the opportunity.
6. _____ Pathogens can often be carried from one person to another.
7. _____ Killing or disabling pathogens on surfaces before they can spread to other people.

    a. Aseptic technique
    b. Person-to-person contact
    c. Opportunistic invasion
    d. Environmental contact
    e. Isolation
    f Disinfection
    g. Sterilization

E. ADDITIONAL ACTIVITY

List 20 Suggested Sanitation Requirements developed from the State of Oregon Model.

1. _____
2. _____
3. _____
4. _____
5. _____
6. _____
7. _____
8. _____
9. _____
10. _____
11. _____
12. _____
13. _____
14. _____

15. _____
16. _____
17. _____
18. _____
19. _____
20. _____

F. PROFESSIONAL APPLICATION

Completing an Accident Report

Most of us recognize that accidents happen daily. When they involve personal injury or property damage, information is needed so that involved parties and any insurance companies can recognize and repair the damages. A massage therapist, like any other business person, may be called upon to fill out an insurance report.

Here is a practice story about an accident. Afterwards, some standard questions, and the correct answers, are supplied, so you can see the way information is to be presented. (Please note that the following scenario is intended to be humorous).

This afternoon, you had a new client. He was the contortionist from the traveling circus, in town for the next week. He brought along his wife, who also works with him, to observe your techniques so she can help him as they travel. Unfortunately, some interesting things happened. You sit for a few minutes to recollect your thoughts, and this is what you remember.

You completed the massage with Mr. Gummy, and had just asked him to roll over when you noticed that the table started swaying. Ms. Gummy, who is an acrobat, was doing a handstand on Mr. Gummy's shoulders. Your table was sturdy enough, but due to the lubricant on your client's shoulders, his wife slid off and out through the window. She was able to catch herself on the awning of the store below yours, but in doing so she bent the frame and tore the canvas. No one was injured, but the other tenant called emergency services, so reports must be filled out.

Since your immediate supervisor was not available, you must fill out the accident report yourself. Using your narrative, fill out the following information for the police and the insurance companies.

1. Where and when did the accident occur?
2. Provide detailed information about the accident.
3. Names and addresses of the person or people involved in the accident.
4. Names of any witnesses to the accident.
5. Names of manufacturers if equipment is involved.
6. Property damage.
7. Physical damage to any people.

ANSWERS:

1. The accident occurred at The Massage Center, 38 Falls Drive, Anytown, ML 48999, on Friday, June 12, 1992, at approximately 11:15 a.m.

2. The incident occurred during a massage therapy session at the above location, in room #4 on the second floor. As I was working with my client, Mr. Victor Gummy, his wife, Ms. Viola Gummy, began doing a handstand on Mr. Gummy's shoulders. Due to the lubricant on his shoulders, Ms. Gummy slid off of Mr. Gummy's shoulders and out through the window. To prevent herself from hitting the sidewalk, Ms. Gummy caught the outer aluminum trim of the front door awning. The awning frame bent and the canvas covering was torn.

3. The people involved in the accident included myself, Cathie Balevit, 38 Falls Drive, Anytown, ML 48999; my client, Victor Gummy; and his wife, Viola Gummy of Fred's Traveling Funshows, 826 Cartwheel Drive, Caravan, FO 81234.

4. Mr. Victor Gummy and I both witnessed Viola Gummy's fall out of the window. Mr. William Bill of Bill's Locksmith Company, 41 Falls Drive, Anytown, ML, actually saw Viola catch herself on the awning as it gave way.

5. The awning was manufactured and installed by Art's Awning Company, 22 Tent Drive, Anytown, ML 48989.

6. The property damage was limited to the awning on the front of the building. An estimate of repair, provided by Art's Awning Company, is attached.

7. There was no damage done to anyone.

Now that you have seen how information needs to be provided, read the following incident narration, and answer the questions that follow.

Today's date is Monday, May 1, 1995. Your client, Mr. James Jackson, arrived for his weekly 4:00 p.m. massage appointment. Twenty minutes into the session, you requested him to roll over from his stomach to his side. As he did so, the table cracked and started to collapse. It did not totally collapse because the cable supports held it up. Other than being a little scared, Mr. Jackson was not injured and you were able to help him off the table. Every Friday you check the tables for safety and do any maintenance. This table was checked and no problems were found.

You immediately contacted the table distributor to tell him of the problem with the table. He works for Buy-Low Products, at 12 Buy-Low Drive in Badtown, VN 84848. He then contacted the manufacturer, Fred's Cut Rate Tables, 480 W. Shady Lane, Market Town, MV 29341. The table is Model #83, called "The Basic," and retails for $99.95.

Please answer the following questions:

1. Where and when did the accident occur?
2. Provide detailed information about the accident.
3. Names and addresses of the person or people involved in the accident.
4. Names of any witnesses to the accident.
5. Names of manufacturers if equipment is involved.
6. Describe all property damage.
7. Detail any physical damage to any and all people involved.

ANSWERS

A. KEY TERMS

1. m
2. a
3. s
4. g
5. e
6. t
7. h
8. r
9. p
10. u
11. b
12. l
13. v
14. c
15. k
16. n
17. o
18. d
19. i
20. j
21. q
22. f

B. FILL IN THE BLANKS

healthy
leading
odors
alcohol

hygiene
sensitive
face
short
covered
uniforms
laundered
contagious

Sanitary
Viruses
Bacteria
Fungi
Yeasts
molds
Protozoa
worms

stop
hand washing
prevent
protect
latex gloves
bleach
soap

hazard

Infants
unattended
minors
pregnancy
assistance
elderly
disabilities

lighting
rugs
uncluttered
traffic
equipment
entrances

non-smoking
metal container
electrical cords
two
open
smoke

C. PUZZLE

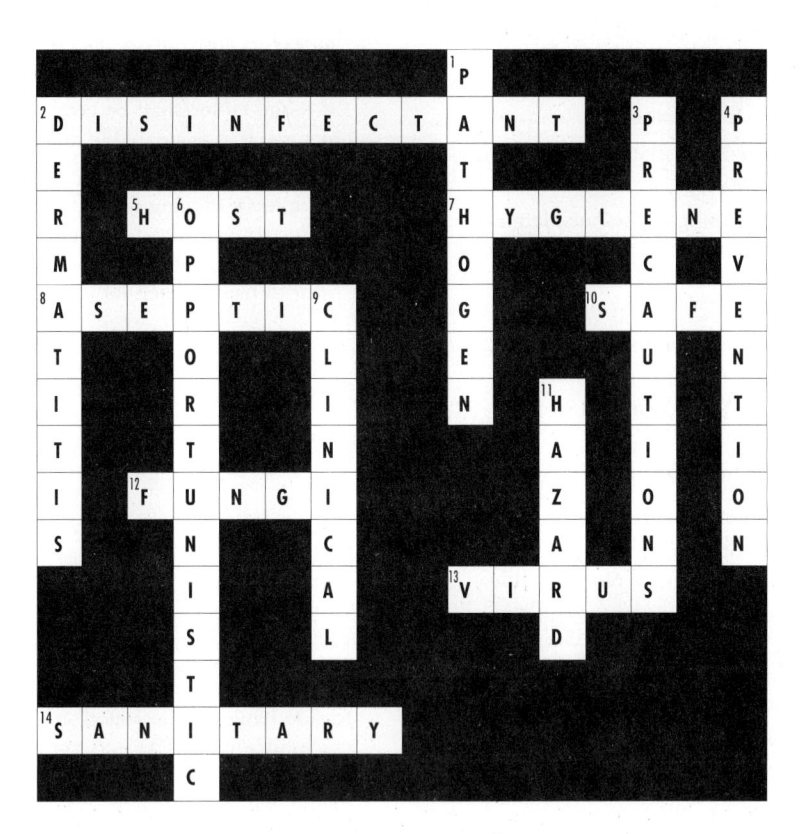

Across:
2. DISINFECTANT
5. HOST
7. HYGIENE
8. ASEPTIC
10. SAFE
12. FUNGI
13. VIRUS
14. SANITARY

Down:
1. PATHOGEN
2. DERMATITIS
3. PRECAUTION (PRCCAUTION — PRECAUTION)
4. PREVENTION
6. OPPORTUNIST
9. CLINICAL
11. HAZARD

D. MATCHING

1. g
2. f
3. e
4. d
5. c
6. b
7. a

E. ADDITIONAL ACTIVITY

1. The massage therapist must clean and wash his or her hands thoroughly with an antibacterial/antiviral agent before contacting each client.
2. The therapist shall wear clean clothing.
3. Lockers or closets for personnel shall be maintained apart from the massage room.
4. All doors and windows opening to the outside air shall be tight-fitting and provision for the exclusion of flies, insects, rodents, or other vermin shall be provided.
5. All floors shall be kept clean, well maintained, and in good repair.
6. Walls and ceilings shall be kept clean and well maintained.
7. Furniture shall be kept clean and in good repair.
8. Have the capability of heating and maintaining room air to a temperature of 75 degrees.
9. Have adequate ventilation to remove objectionable odors.
10. Have lighting fixtures capable of providing a minimum of five foot candles of light at floor level; they shall be used during cleaning operation.
11. All sewage and liquid waste shall be disposed of in a municipal sewage system or an approved septic system.
12. The water supply shall be adequate, deemed safe by the health department, and sanitary.
13. Drinking fountains of an approved type or individual paper drinking cups shall be provided.
14. Every massage business shall be provided with a sanitary toilet facility with an adequate supply of hot and cold water under pressure and shall be conveniently located for use by the employees and patrons.
15. Toilet room doors shall be tightly fitting and the rooms shall be kept clean, in good repair, and free from flies, insects, and vermin.
16. A supply of soap in a covered dispenser and single-use sanitary towels in a dispenser shall be provided at each lavatory installation with a covered waste receptacle for proper disposal.
17. A supply of toilet paper on a dispenser shall be available for each toilet installation.
18. Massage lubricants including but not limited to oil, soap, alcohol, powders, and lotions, shall be dispensed from suitable containers to be used and stored in such a manner as to prevent contamination.
19. Any unused lubricant coming into physical contact with the client or the massage therapist must be disposed.
20. Use only freshly laundered sheets and linens.
21. All soiled (used) linens washed in a mechanical clothes washing machine which provides a hot water temperature of at least 140 degrees Fahrenheit and subject to antiviral agents (10% bleach solution, i.e., nine parts water to one part bleach).
22. Massage tables shall be covered with impervious material that is cleanable and shall be kept clean and in good repair.
23. Equipment coming in contact with the client shall be thoroughly cleansed with soap or other suitable detergent and water followed by adequate sanitation prior to use on each individual client.

F. PROFESSIONAL APPLICATION

ANSWERS

1. The accident occurred on Monday, May 1, 1995, at approximately 4:20 p.m. (List your clinic name and address here).

2. My client was receiving a massage during his weekly session. I requested that he turn from a prone position to side-lying. As he rolled to his side, we both heard a cracking sound. The massage table surface then partially collapsed downward. It was kept from fully giving way by the cable supports. The client was uninjured and able to climb off the table with some assistance.

   The massage table had been checked on Friday, April 28, 1995, as part of a weekly routine maintenance and safety check. No problems were found at that time.

3. I was working as the therapist. My name is (fill in your name and full address). The client was Mr. James Jackson (fill in his full name and address from your client information form).

   NOTE: It is always a good idea to provide phone numbers even if they are not requested.

4. The witnesses were myself and Mr. Jackson.

5. The table was Model #83, "The Basic," with a retail price of $99.95. It is manufactured by Fred's Cut Rate Tables, 480 W. Shady Lane, in Market Town, MV 29341. It was sold to me by Buy-Low Products of 12 Buy-Low Drive, Badtown, VN 84848.

6. The property damage was limited to the table. The top surface is split, both the wood and the vinyl covering, the outer supports are cracked, and the hinge is bent. An estimate of repair costs will be forwarded when received.

7. No physical damage was done to anyone.

ADDITIONAL NOTE: Since the client was involved, he will be requested to provide information. You must still have his written permission to provide his name, address, and phone number since you were providing a service to him and have guaranteed confidentiality.

CHAPTER 6

The Scientific Art

A. KEY TERMS

Match the term to the best definition.

1. autoregulation _____
2. body/mind _____
3. centering _____
4. cognitive _____
5. counterirritation _____
6. endogenous _____
7. endorphin _____
8. feedback _____
9. gate control theory _____
10. hardening _____
11. hyperstimulation analgesia _____
12. intuition _____
13. law _____
14. nerve impingement _____
15. noxious _____
16. placebo _____
17. reflex _____
18. science _____
19. somatic _____
20. subtle energies _____

a. The ability to focus on a specific circumstance through screening sensation.
b. Superficial stimulation that relieves deeper sensation by stimulation of different sensory signals.
c. Weak electrical fields that are said to surround and run through the body.
d. An involuntary response to a stimulus. Reflexes are specific, predictable, adaptive, and purposeful.
e. The interaction between thought and physiology connected to the limbic system, hypothalamus influence of the autonomic nervous system, and the endocrine system.
f. Unpleasant.
g. A scientific statement that is found to be true for a whole class of natural occurrences.
h. A method of teaching the body to deal more effectively with stress.
i. A method of autoregulation to maintain internal homeostasis that interlinks body functions.
j. Made in the body.
k. Part of the endogenous opioid peptides that have morphine-like analgesic properties, behavioral effects, and neurotransmitter and neuromodulator functions.

l. Reduction of perception of a sensation by stimulation of large-diameter nerve fibers.

m. Awareness with perception, reasoning, judgement, intuition, and memory.

n. Knowing something by using subconscious information.

o. Hypothesis that painful stimuli may be prevented from reaching higher levels of the central nervous system by stimulation of larger sensory nerves.

p. Pressure against a nerve by skin, fascia, muscles, ligaments, and joints.

q. A treatment for an illness that influences the course of the disease even if the treatment is not specifically validated.

r. Pertaining to the body.

s. The intellectual process to understand by observation, measurement, accumulation of data, and analysis of the findings.

t. Control of homeostasis by alteration of tissue or function.

B. FILL IN THE BLANKS

_____ is defined as the intellectual process for using all of the mental and physical resources available in order to better understand, explain, and predict normal as well as unusual natural phenomena. _____ is defined as knowing something without going through a rational process of thinking. _____ is the ability to pay attention to, or focus on a specific area. Centering is the skill to screen sensation and the ability to concentrate.

Massage is _____ sensory stimulation. The fundamental concepts of the effects of therapeutic massage can be broken down into two categories: _____ methods that directly affect the soft tissue through techniques that normalize the connective tissue or move body fluids and intestinal contents, and _____ methods that stimulate the nervous system, chemical system, and endocrine system.

Effective bodywork is achieved through massage methods interacting with the _____. The _____ quality of massage complicates the research issue because of the complexity of human beings and the interaction of the client practitioner dynamics that have effects on the results of massage. Because of technologic advances, the validation for massage can be more _____ based on scientific methods instead of subjective observation from experiential evidence.

Responses and effects of massage on the nervous system are _____. The nervous system is divided into the _____ nervous system, consisting of the brain, spinal cord and coverings, and the _____ nervous system, which consists of nerves and ganglions. The peripheral nervous system is further divided into the _____ and somatic divisions. The autonomic division is subdivided into the sympathetic and _____ systems. The influence of the nervous system _____ the endocrine system and neurochemicals. The feedback system and _____ (maintaining of internal homeostasis) is interlinked with all body functions. The stimulation of the body by massage influences the autonomic nervous system and _____ system response. The limbic system is a group of brain structures activated by _____ behavior and arousal that influences the endocrine and autonomic systems. The _____ controls subconscious movements of skeletal muscle, input from proprioceptors, feedback loops, posture, future positioning, and regulates sensations of anger and pleasure. Research indicates that the cerebellum, the limbic pain and pleasure centers, and the various relay centers are all part of one _____. _____ is the superficial irritation that relieves irritation of deeper structures. Counterirritation may be explained by Malzack and Wall's _____ Theory. Reduction of pain by _____, using massage and acupuncture, has been used for many years.

It is common to have soft tissue _____ on nerves. Because of the structural arrangement of the body, these impingements often occur at major _____ plexuses. If the _____ plexus is being impinged, the person will experience headaches, neck pain, and breathing difficulties.

The_____ plexus is situated partly in the neck and partly in the axilla and provides virtually all the nerves that innervate the upper limb. _____ plexus nerve impingement may give rise to low back discomfort with a belt distribution of pain, lower abdominal pain, genital pain, thigh pain, and medial lower leg pain.

The _____ plexus has about a dozen named branches with the main branch being the sciatic nerve. Input from the sensory systems plays a role in control of _____ functions by stimulating spinal reflex mechanisms. Methods of massage that use _____ touch stimulate root hair plexus, free nerve endings, Merkel's discs (tactile), Meissner's corpuscles (touch), and end organs of Ruffini (cutaneous mechanoreceptor). Techniques such as compression, deep gliding strokes, and joint movement stimulate the _____ receptors known as Pacinian corpuscles (lamellated) and type II cutaneous mechanoreceptors. Rapid and repetitive sensory signals of _____ and _____ techniques directly influence the corpuscles of touch and the Pacinian corpuscles (lamellated). Therapeutic massage introduces touch, pressure, vibration and positional stimuli, causing _____ receptor neurons to respond. Movement, stretch, and pressure methods of massage focus the effects of these activities on the muscles, tendons, joints, and ligaments to stimulate the _____.

_____ are fast, predictable, automatic responses to a change in the environment and help to maintain homeostasis. Therapeutic massage stimulation constitutes a _____ in the environment. The reflexes most often stimulated are the_____ reflex, tendon reflex, flexor reflex, and crossed extensor reflex. The stretch reflex is activated by the muscle _____, which sense muscle stretching. The _____ reflex operates as a feedback mechanism to control muscle tension by causing muscle relaxation. The flexor (withdrawal) and crossed extensor reflexes are_____ reflex arcs. When these reflexes are stimulated, _____ sides of the body are affected through intersegmental reflex arcs. The _____ reflex is involved in moving away from a stimuli, and the _____ reflex is involved in maintaining balance. It is important that the receptor being targeted is accessed with the appropriate technique and _____, so that the reflex stimulated is allowed to function in the appropriate manner.

Activation of the _____ nervous system usually results in sensations that people call stress. When we become fatigued, _____ functions signal for rest. There is exciting, ongoing research concerning _____ learning in the areas of sympathetic and parasympathetic patterns of function. Breathing is a powerful way to interact with the_____ nervous system. Chest breathing and _____ are common components of increased sympathetic stimulation. Toughening/hardening is the repeated exposure to stimuli that elicit _____ responses. Like exercise, _____ methods using active participation of the client help to dissipate (burn off) sympathetic stress hormones (sympathoadrenal response), allowing the system to reestablish _____.

There are several endogenous opiate-like compounds within the body, including _____ and beta-endorphins. Some methods of massage depend on the _____ of a moderate controlled pain to relieve pain. Negative feedback system that activates the release of serotonin and opiates which _____ pain. The effects of these and other _____ released during massage may explain and validate the use of sensory stimulation methods for chronic pain, anxiety, and depression. It is possible that the gentle, caring attention focused on the client during therapeutic massage interacts with the powerful and important_____ effect.

Other approaches to the fascial or connective tissue component of muscles are called _____ techniques. All the _____ in the body is directly linked together like a three dimensional body stocking. Massage that provides for a gentle sustained _____ on the fascial component will affect this type of connective tissue. Travell and Simons, and others suggest that the effects of massage on the myofascial _____ are from the stimulation of proprioceptive nerve endings, the release of enkephalin, the stretch of musculotendinous structures that initiate reflex muscle relaxation through the Golgi tendon organ and spindle receptors, and increased circulation.

Increases in the blood and lymph circulation are the most widely recognized of the _____ effects of massage therapy. Increased blood flow on a local level is achieved by _____ of tissues, which empties venous beds and lowers venous pressure and increases capillary blood flow that is quickly counteracted by _____. Massage stimulates the release of _____, especially histamine. Compression against arteries will _____ influence the internal pressure receptors in the arteries. Therapeutic massage could play an important role in _____ programs by providing a natural mechanism to stimulate the body to adjust to the stress of daily life and restore the natural homeostatic balance. The massage professional can provide the services of this art and be confident that there are _____ reasons for why massage works and feels good.

C. PUZZLE

Fill in the spaces with the following words:

analgesia

autoregulation

cognitive

counterirritation

endogenous

endorphin

feedback

impingement

intuition

placebo

reflex

somatic

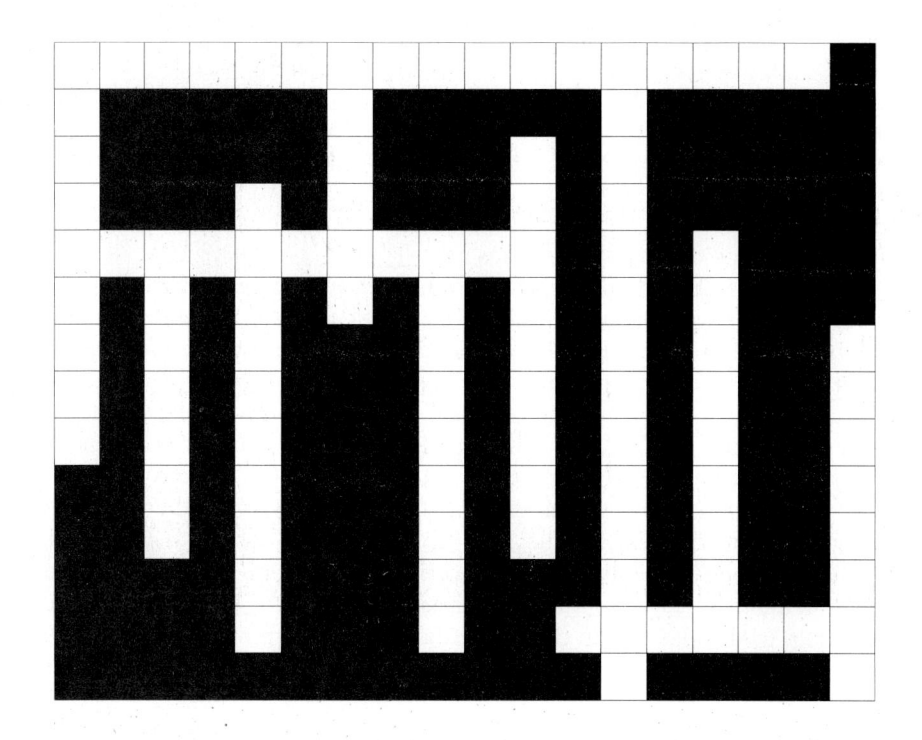

D. LABELING

Label the major nerve plexuses for Figure 6.1.

brachial plexus
brain
cervical plexus
lumbar plexus
nerves
sacral plexus
spinal cord

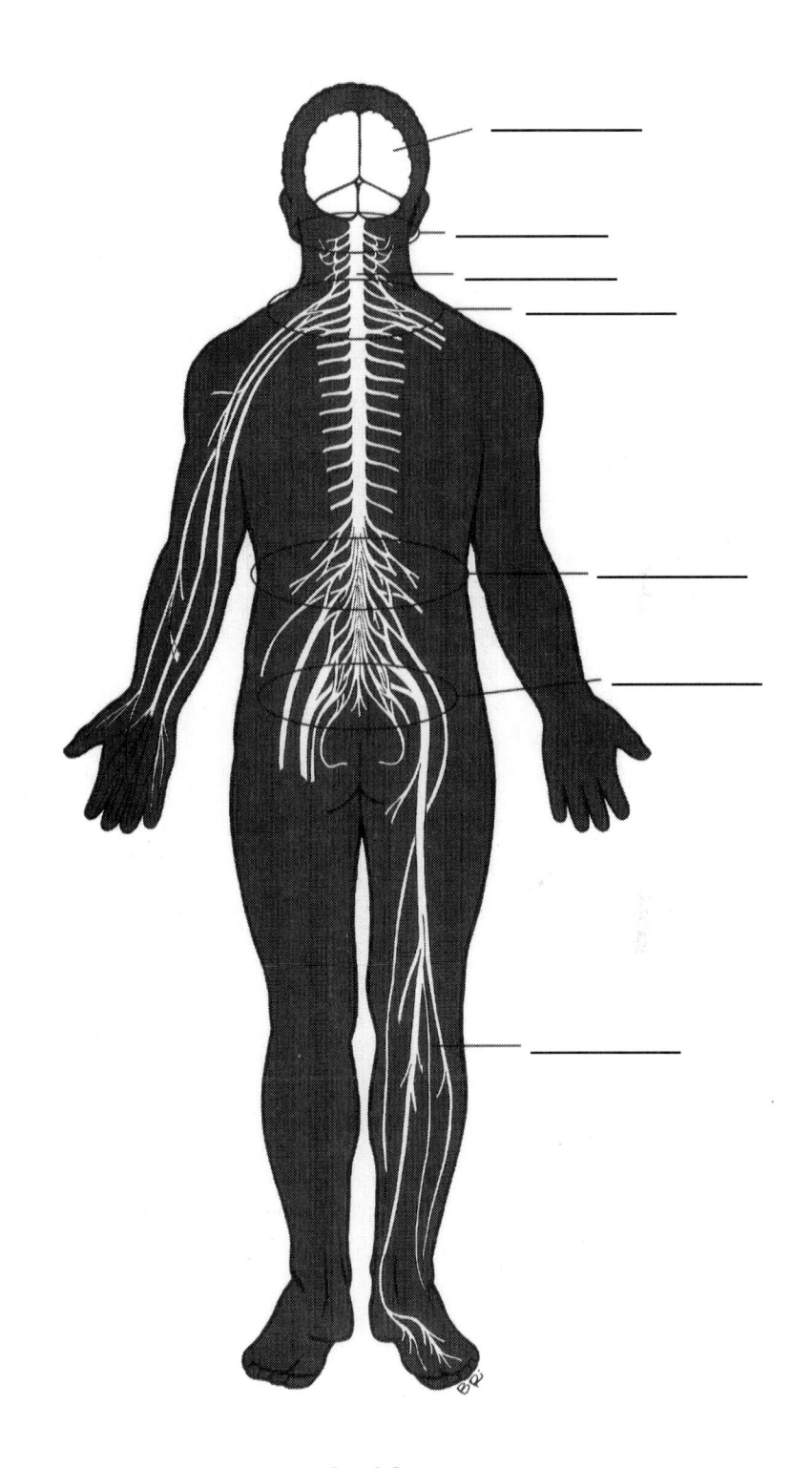

Fig. 6.1

E. MATCHING

a. Match the scientific laws affecting massage with their descriptions.

1. ____ The weakest stimulus capable of producing a response produces the maximum response contraction in cardiac and skeletal muscle and nerves.

2. ____ Anterior spinal nerve roots are motor and posterior spinal nerve roots are sensory.

3. ____ When an impulse has passed once through a certain set of neurons to the exclusion of others, it will tend to take the same course on a future occasion, and each time it transverses this path the resistance will be smaller.

4. ____ The stress used to stretch or compress a body is proportional to the strain as long as the elastic limits of the body have not been exceeded.

5. ____ Excitation of a receptor always gives rise to the same sensation regardless of the nature of the stimulus.

6. ____ The increase in stimulus necessary to produce the smallest perceptible increase in sensation bears a constant ratio to the strength of the stimulus already acting.

7. ____ A nerve trunk which supplies a joint also supplies the muscles of the joint and the skin over the insertions of such muscles.

8. ____ If a mild irritation is applied to one or more sensory nerves, the movement will take place usually on one side only, and that side which is irritated.

9. ____ If the stimulation is sufficiently increased, motor reaction is manifested, not only by the irritated side, but also in similar muscles on the opposite side of the body.

10. ____ Reflex movements are usually more intense on the side of irritation; at times, the movements of the opposite side equal them in intensity, but they are usually less pronounced.

11. ____ If the excitation continues to increase, it is propagated upward, and reactions take place through centrifugal nerves coming from the cord segments higher up.

12. ____ When the irritation becomes very intense, it is propagated in the medulla oblongata, which becomes a focus from which stimuli radiate to all parts of the cord, causing a general contraction of all muscles to the body.

13. ____ Weak stimuli activate physiologic processes; very strong stimuli inhibit them.

14. ____ When autonomic effectors are partially or completely separated from their normal nerve connections, they become more sensitive to the action of chemical substances.

a. Hilton's Law
b. Law of Unilaterality
c. Law of Facilitation
d. Hooke's Law
e. Law of Generalization
f. Arndt-Schultz Law
g. All-or-None or Bowditch's Law
h. Bell's Law
i. Law of Specificity of Nervous Energy
j. Weber's Law
k. Law of Symmetry
l. Law of Intensity
m. Law of Radiation
n. Cannon's Law of Denervation

b. *Match the visceral functions with their sympathetic or parasympathetic controls.*

Column 1 contains the visceral function. Choosing the best response from the control list below, place the corresponding letter in Column 2. In Column 3, write either an S for Sympathetic or a P for Parasympathetic, depending on the control response.

Column 1	Column 2	Column 3
1. heart muscle	_____	_____
2. digestive tract	_____	_____
3. skeletal muscle blood vessels	_____	_____
4. smooth muscle blood vessels	_____	_____
5. urinary bladder	_____	_____
6. iris of eye	_____	_____
7. pilomotor muscles	_____	_____
8. adrenal medulla	_____	_____
9. sweat glands	_____	_____
10. digestive glands	_____	_____

Column 2 Control List - enter letter from list below in Column 2 above.

a. increases secretion of digestive juices

b. increases sweat secretion

c. slows heartbeat

d. constricts blood vessels

e. relaxes bladder

f. increases peristalsis

g. dilates blood vessels

h. increases epinephrine secretion

i. stimulates goose pimples

j. constricts pupil

F. PROBLEM SOLVING EXERCISES

1. A client is referred by the physician to you for basic relaxation massage to ease chronic pain of undetermined cause. Using information presented in Chapter 6, list at least four principle reasons why the massage could benefit the client.

   _____
   _____
   _____
   _____

2. A client experiences a reduction in anxiety and impatience after receiving a series of massages. How would you explain this?

   _____
   _____
   _____
   _____

G. PROFESSIONAL APPLICATION

1. Make a list of your daily experiences with autonomic nervous system functions. Make a second list of those autonomic functions that you encounter while doing massage.

   _____
   _____
   _____
   _____

2. Read through the various therapeutic massage journals. Find one or two articles regarding bodywork and classify the information presented by the following effects.

   a. classify methods as mechanical or reflexive
   b. classify if primary systemic effect is the nervous system and within the nervous system somatic, visceral, peripheral, central or autonomic. connective tissue, circulation
   c. identify what chemical (i.e., hormone) and neurotransmitters are being stimulated
   d. identify the sensory receptor responsible for responding to the stimulation

H. RESEARCH FOR FURTHER STUDY

Design a possible research study. Develop an idea (hypothesis), narrow the topic, then decide what measurements will be used. Identify possible outcomes. Identity what other things may influence the outcome. Look at other research for examples of research design patterns. Locate resources for how to develop a research study.

_____
_____
_____
_____
_____
_____
_____
_____
_____

ANSWERS

1. KEY TERMS

1. t
2. e
3. a
4. m
5. b
6. j
7. k
8. i
9. o
10. h
11. l
12. n
13. g
14. p
15. f
16. q
17. d
18. s
19. r
20. c

B. FILL IN THE BLANKS

Science
Intuition
Centering

external
mechanical
reflexive

physiology
subjective
objective

reflexive
central
peripheral
autonomic
parasympathetic
regulates
autoregulation
limbic
emotional
cerebellum
circuit
Counterirritation
Gate Control
hyperstimulation analgesia

impinging
nerve
cervical

brachial
Lumbar

sacral
motor
light
pressure
vibration
percussion
sensory
proprioceptors

Reflexes
change
stretch
spindles
tendon
polysynaptic
both
flexor
crossed extensor
intensity

sympathetic
parasympathetic
state dependent
autonomic
hyperventilation
arousal
massage
homeostasis

enkephalin
creation
inhibit
neurotransmitters
placebo

myofascial
fascia
pull
trigger points

physiologic
compression
autoregulation
vasodilators
mechanically
prevention
scientific

C. PUZZLE

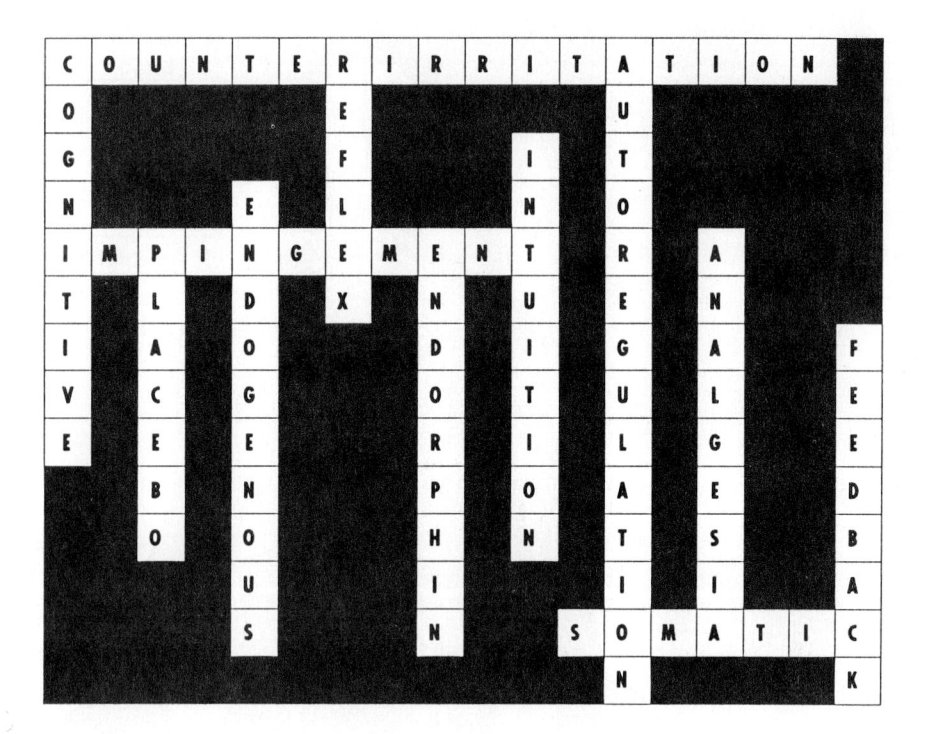

The Scientific Art

Across:
- COUNTERIRRITATION
- IMPINGEMENT
- SOMATIC

Down:
- COGNITIVE
- PLACEBO
- ENDOGENOUS
- REFLEX
- ENDORPHIN
- INTUITION
- AUTOREGULATION
- ANALGESICS
- SOMATIZATION
- FEEDBACK

D. LABELING

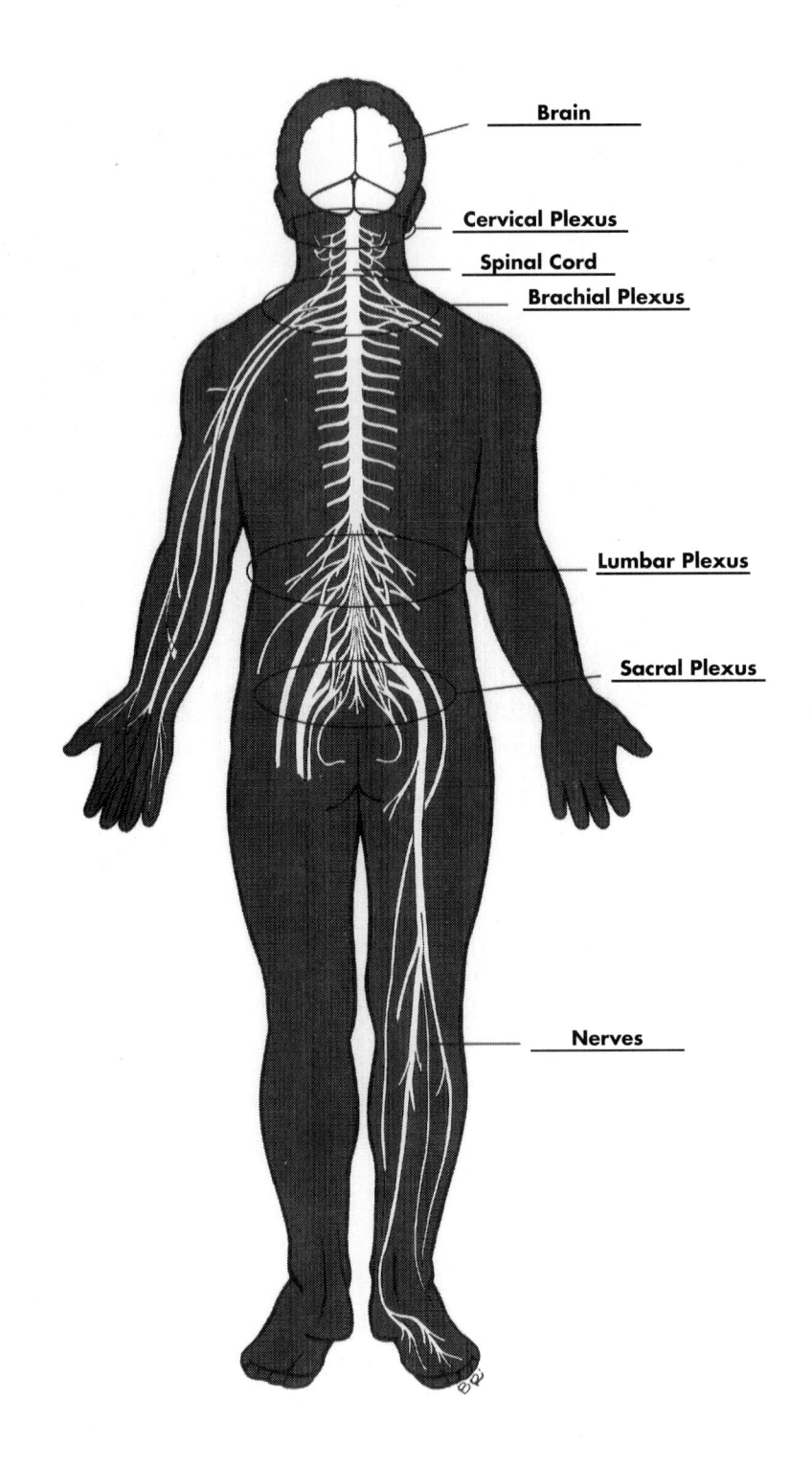

- Brain
- Cervical Plexus
- Spinal Cord
- Brachial Plexus
- Lumbar Plexus
- Sacral Plexus
- Nerves

E. MATCHING

a.
1. g
2. h
3. c
4. d
5. i
6. j
7. a
8. b
9. k
10. l
11. m
12. e
13. f
14. n

b.
1. c   P
2. f   P
3. g   S
4. d   S
5. e   S
6. j   P
7. i   S
8. h   S
9. b   S
10. a P

F. PROBLEM SOLVING EXERCISES

1.
counterirritation
hyperstimulation analgesia
release of endorphins and serotonin
hardening
placebo effect

2.
reduction of sympathetic arousal responses
increased ability to restore homeostasis
increased energy due to reduced generalized muscle tension
increased circulation provides for all over increase in efficient functioning
restoration of effective parasympathetic restorative function

CHAPTER 7

Business and Professional Practice Management

A. KEY TERMS

Match the term to the best definition.

1. brochure _____
2. burn-out _____
3. business plan _____
4. client-practitioner agreement and policy statement _____
5. employee _____
6. fees _____
7. goal _____
8. marketing _____
9. management _____
10. media _____
11. motivation _____
12. paper trail _____
13. resume _____
14. self-employed _____
15. start-up costs _____
16. zoning _____

a. A projection for business development.
b. All activities that are required to maintain a business, particularly record keeping and financial dispersement.
c. Informational sources of television, radio, print (newspaper, magazine etc.).
d. The internal drive that provides the energy to do what is necessary to accomplish a goal.
e. Charges for services provided (rendered).
f. A short educational document that explains the services offered, qualifications of practitioner, fees, etc.
g. A detailed, written explanation of all rules, expectations, and procedures for the massage.
h. The organization and documentation in writing of all business activities.
i. A projected achievement that can be accomplished in a relatively short period of time.

j. A summary of professional experiences and qualifications.

k. One who works for one's self.

l. Using up energy faster than it is replenished, often from taking care of others more than we take care of ourselves.

m. Money required to begin a business and continue support until the business is viable.

n. Advertising and other promotional activities to sell a product or service.

o. A local government regulation of land use.

p. One who works for another person.

B. FILL IN THE BLANKS

To succeed at anything one must be _____. Therapeutic massage is the _____ as any other business. It is important to market the _____ — your skills as a massage practitioner, and to attend to the record keeping and financial commitments required of the business person. Even if the practitioner chooses to be an _____ rather than a self-employed professional, it is important to understand the obligations and time _____ required of the employer.

A professional should plan to give a new business _____ years of constant attention for it to grow from strong roots and a solid foundation. It will be about _____ years before attention to the business can be relaxed and small portions of it entrusted to another supervising person for short periods of time. With all the possibilities available to the massage practitioner, it will be necessary eventually to _____ the focus to one, two, or three specific markets so that advertising and promotional activities are_____.

Each business person needs a diverse group of _____ people, including a _____, an accountant or skilled bookkeeper, an advertising-marketing consultant, and an advisor for business planning. Experience is truly the best teacher, and we learn from our _____ and our successes. Self-esteem is very _____ to successful business practices. _____ occurs when you use your energy up faster than you can restore it.

A _____ is a professional and personal summary of a person. Development of the _____ begins in school. _____ are important because they provide direction and _____ for achievement. _____ are the initial expenses of beginning a business. _____ is the advertising and other promotional activities required to sell a product or service. The _____ is the primary tool to educate the public and potential clients concerning the services being offered. _____ advertising (newspaper, radio, and television) is very expensive and not the best idea initially. When considering money and how much to charge for a service, it is important to realize that people usually live life based on an equal exchange for services rendered or for goods received. This is called the _____.

The most common type of massage practitioner is the _____ massage therapist. It is also important to remember that the self-employed massage therapist must figure _____, which is the amount actually put into the business. At a minimum, for every hour spent giving a massage, at least an _____ will be spent with business work such as records, clean-up, advertising, and marketing. When all the pros and cons are considered, the salary ends up being about the _____, whether the practitioner is an employee of someone at an hourly wage, or owns his or her own business.

_____ includes all the activities that are required to maintain a business particularly record keeping and financial dispersement. It is _____ to have the client read a client-practitioner agreement and policy statement. This booklet is more _____ than the brochure. This process becomes part of the _____ process. The agreement or policy statement provides the practitioner with an opportunity to _____ the practice.

C. PUZZLE

Unscramble the following words to find terms used in this chapter:

1. crebhour _____
2. truboun _____
3. pleeyemo _____
4. sefe _____
5. loga _____
6. grametink _____
7. tanemagmen _____
8. deima _____
9. vimanitoto _____
10. esmeru _____
11. gonzin _____

D. ADDITIONAL ACTIVITY

When developing a client-practitioner agreement and policy statement, you need to be specific regarding certain areas of information provided. With each of the sections presented, put in the valid information that a client will need to know. When you are done, you will have a comprehensive outline to use in creating the booklet.

Use Box 7.4 (pp. 170-172) in the text as a guideline for the information needed. For example, in Section 1, the text says to explain what type of work you provide. You are to list either therapeutic massage, reflexology, or whatever it is that you do.

Some of the answers for this section are samples you can use to compare your responses; others are a reiteration of the information which you will need to detail.

Client Practitioner Agreement and Policy Statement
All entries should be specific as to the following items:

1. The nature of the service offered:

    a. _____

    b. _____

    c. _____

    d. _____

2. Description of the service offered:

   a. _____

   b. _____

   c. _____

   d. _____

3. Qualifications of the practitioner:

   a. _____

   b. _____

4. Client financial and time investment:

   a. _____

   b. _____

   c. _____

   d. _____

   e. _____

5. Role of the client in health care:

   a. _____

   b. _____

6. Type of service:

   a. _____

   b. _____

   c. _____

   d. _____

   e. _____

7. Training and experience:

   a. _____

   b. _____

   c. _____

   d. _____

   e. _____

8. Appointment policies:

   a. _____

   b. _____

   c. _____

   d. _____

   e. _____

9. Client/Practitioner expectations and informed consent:
   a.
   b.
   c.
   d.
   e.
   f.
   g.
   h.
   i.

10. Fees:
    a.
    b.
    c.
    d.
    e.
    f.
    g.
    h.
    i.

11. Sexual appropriateness:

    a. _____

    b. _____

12. Recourse policy:

    a. _____

    b. _____

E. PROBLEM SOLVING EXERCISES

1. Tom is notified that a client is unhappy with his massage fees and is considering finding another massage professional with lower fees. What steps can Tom take to support his fee structure?

2. Marilyn is having a meeting with a client who she feels may have difficulty with understanding the scope of practice of massage. How can she use the client-practitioner agreement and policy statement booklet to help establish professional boundaries and provide informed consent?

3. Calculate real time required to learn massage.

4. Terry begins a private massage practice after graduation from school. She follows all the recommendations in the business section, business begins to build slowly but then levels off. Word of mouth advertising is not working as well as expected. What steps can Terry take to boost business?

___

F. PROFESSIONAL APPLICATION

1. A client calls about receiving massage. You speak with her on the phone and offer to send her your client policies and procedures booklet. After two weeks you do not hear from the prospective client. You call as a follow-up and the client has specific questions about certain aspects of the policy booklet. This client tells you that a previous massage therapist did not have all these rules. What would you do?

___

2. Motivation Statement

   In the space below list three things that motivate you to become a massage practitioner.

___

3. Define the following items as they relate directly to you.

Know thyself ___

Follow your dream ___

WIIFM ___

Whatever we believe with emotion and feeling becomes our reality ___

Believe in your product ___

Provide a quality product ___

4. Develop personal application of methods to prevent "burn-out." Call it "The Burnout Plan," or some other clever name. List one idea for each of these areas:

Care of physical needs _____
Support person _____
Care of spiritual needs _____
Continuing education _____
Get-away time _____

5. The business structure of therapeutic massage takes many forms. There is a difference between the massage employee and the self-employed massage professional. Choose which approach you plan to pursue and list those areas of the chapter that most pertain to your professional development plan.

6. List five business goals. Use the five recommendations for goal setting in Box 7.2 in the text as a guide. Box 7.2 is condensed for your convenience and follows:

Hints for setting goals:
1. State goals in the present tense.
2. Make sure your goals are realistic and attainable.
3. Speak in the positive.
4. Set target deadlines for yourself.
5. Make sure your goals are small steps toward your ultimate plan.

In each goal, circle any portion that meets the first recommendation.
Underline any portion that meets the second recommendation.
Put a box around any portion that meets the third recommendation.
Double underline any portion that meets the fourth recommendation.
Double circle any portion that meets the fifth recommendation.

Sample:

⬚(I will)⬚ (1,3) ⦅complete this exercise⦆ (2,5) within the next thirty minutes (4).

_____
_____
_____
_____
_____

G. RESEARCH FOR FURTHER STUDY

1. Compare the business procedures outlined in the text to another business operation and identify both similarities and differences in those procedures.

_____
_____
_____
_____

2. The statement "Business is Business" is applicable to massage. List resources in your area for further business education such as community college courses, chamber of commerce, etc.

_____
_____
_____
_____

ANSWERS

A. KEY TERMS

1. f
2. l
3. a
4. g
5. p
6. e
7. i
8. n
9. b
10. c
11. d
12. h
13. j
14. k
15. m
16. o

B. FILL IN THE BLANKS

motivated
same
product
employee
commitments

two
five
narrow
manageable

support
lawyer
mistakes
important
Burnout

resume
business plan
Goals
landmarks
Start up costs
Marketing
brochure
Media
equity hypothesis

self-employed
real time
hour
same

Management
essential
comprehensive
informed consent
define

C. PUZZLE

1. brochure
2. burnout
3. employee
4. fees
5. goal
6. marketing
7. management
8. media
9. motivation
10. resume
11. zoning

D. ADDITIONAL ACTIVITY

1. The nature of the service offered:
   a. Clearly explain that therapeutic massage is a general health service.
   b. State that no specific treatment of any kind is given for pre-existing physical or mental problems.
   c. Referrals will be made to the appropriate licensed professional for specific medical, structural, psychological, or dietary nature problems.
   d. Written permission and supervision by the medical or other licensed health professional will be required to work with any conditions which fall within their scope of practice.

2. Description of the service offered:
   a. (Include a full description of the types of services offered and the procedures followed in rendering those services.)
   b. Clients may remain dressed and will always be properly draped.
   c. The client may stop the session at anytime and may choose not to have any area of their body touched or any particular techniques used.
   d. (Simply explain the process of a massage.)

3. Qualifications of the practitioner:
   a. (List verifiable credentials documenting the education, training, licensing, certifications, and experience to allow potential clients to verify, for themselves, the accuracy and competency of the practitioner.)
   b. (List the organization issuing the credentials, such as a school or continuing education provider.)

4. Client financial and time investment:
   a. Include a realistic statement of costs and fees in the brochure.
   b. Emphasize that the effects of massage are temporary and massage is best used as a maintenance system.
   c. Indicate that the effects of the massage session can be increased with simple exercises. The massage practitioner will teach self-help to the client if requested.
   d. The best results from massage are maintained when implemented on a weekly or biweekly bases.
   e. Therapeutic massage, when used occasionally, will only provide temporary effects.

5. Role of the client in health care:
   a. Include the importance of the client responsibility in personal health care.
   b. It is important for the client to realize that the role of the massage therapist as a facilitator in the wellness process.

6. Type of service:
   a. Our clinic offers relaxation, prenatal, and sports massages.
   b. Explain what this particular style of bodywork is good for and what are its limitations.
   c. Specify if you specialize in working with any particular group, such as the elderly, athletes, or with specific problems like headaches and back pain.
   d. Indicate if there are certain situations that you do not care to work with, such as pregnant women or people with certain medical conditions.
   e. Have a referral network of related professionals that you use.

7. Training and experience:
   a. Licensing information. Does your state require licensing? If so, have the facts confirming that you are licensed available.
   b. State how long you have been in practice, what school you attended, if the school was approved by any professional organization, and how many classroom hours were required for graduation.
   c. Provide information regarding continuing education.
   d. Provide additional education if pertinent (i.e., that you are also an athletic trainer).
   e. Include the names of any professional affiliations of which you are an active member.

8. Appointment policies:
   a. Define the length of an average session.
   b. Inform clients which days you work, your hours, and if you do on-site work, either residential or business.
   c. Tell the client to expect that the first appointment will be longer than subsequent appointments, whether or not you take emergency appointments, and how often you suggest clients come for a massage session.
   d. Be clear with the cancellation policy and your policy for late appointments.

e. Explain to the client whether to eat before an appointment, or if physical activity should be altered or restricted before or after the session.

9. Client/Practitioner expectations and informed consent:
   a. Explain in detail what happens at the first bodywork session (i.e., paperwork, medical history, etc.).
   b. Clients should know that they can get partially undressed, or undressed down to their shorts or panties, and that clients are covered and draped during the session.
   c. Explain the order in which you massage (face up or face down to begin), what parts of the body you work on and in what order, if you use oils, if a shower is available before or after the massage or if bathing at home before attending the massage appointment is expected.
   d. Make sure the client understands if talking is appropriate during the session and that you should be informed if anything feels uncomfortable.
   e. If you have low lighting and music is provided, the client should be comfortable with that aspect of the massage.
   f. Make clear to the client the possibility of any reactions that may be expected.
   g. Indicate that the goals for the massage session and proposed styles and massage methods will be discussed with the client prior to the massage and that consent will need to be provided for all massage procedures.
   h. Inform the client that your profession has a code of ethics and indicate your policy on confidentiality.
   i. If the client is in any way uncomfortable, it is permissible to be accompanied by a friend or relative.

10. Fees:
    a. fees are reviewed annually, and any increases will begin in April.
    b. a sliding fee is available for retirees, those on disability, etc.
    c. cash, check, and major credit cards are acceptable for payment.
    d. payment is expected at time of service; any arrangements for billing must be made in advance.
    e. clients are responsible for collecting from insurance.
    f. insurance covers our services only when client is referred by physician and has written pre-approval from insurance company.
    g. our fees are based on hourly rates.
    h. a 20% discount is offered to all clients who purchase a series of 5 sessions.
    i. to thank you for referring new clients to our office, we offer you a $5 discount on your next session.

11. Sexual appropriateness:
    a. Sexual behavior by the therapist toward the client and the client toward the therapist is always unethical and inappropriate.
    b. It is always the responsibility of the therapist or health professional to see that sexual misconduct does not occur.

12. Recourse policy:
    a. If a client is unhappy or dissatisfied, a portion of the fees will be refunded.
    b. If the matter is not handled in a satisfactory manner, clients can contact the Organization of Bodyworkers of Tylerville to register any complaints.

E. PROBLEM SOLVING EXERCISES

1. Determine fees charged by other therapists in the surrounding area. Locate information about education levels and cost comparable to his that may validate higher fees.

2. Send booklet to clients to read before massage. Use booklet as a guide of carefully thought out policies when interviewing the client.

3. Take into account the following and then total:
   Time in school
   Time spent commuting to school
   Time spent completing homework
   Time spent doing research
   Time devoted to practical practice

4.
   a. Talk with current clients about their satisfaction with your service and ask if they are referring new clients.
   b. Consider offering incentives for referrals.
   c. Take continuing education and advertise about your new skills.
   d. Do a direct mail with a special offer to current clients.
   e. Volunteer to work at some special events.

F. PROFESSIONAL APPLICATION

1. Offer to have the client come in and talk with you.

    Identify the areas of concern for the client and expand on the information in the booklet.

    Explain the professional aspects of informed consent.

    Explain that knowledge and clarity on these aspects supports the professional relationship.

CHAPTER 8

Body Mechanics

A. KEY TERMS

Match the term to the best definition.

1. asymmetrical stance _____
2. body mechanics _____
3. compressive force _____
4. symmetrical stance _____

   a. Use of the body in an efficient and biomechanically correct way.
   b. Pressure focused in a particular direction.
   c. Position in which the body weight is distributed equally between the feet.
   d. Position in which the body weight is shifted from one foot to the other during standing.

B. FILL IN THE BLANKS

_____ allow the practitioner's body to be used in a careful, efficient, and deliberate way. Efficient use of the body will help to prevent _____. Massage therapy has unique _____ and physical demands. Injury will result if the massage professional is not careful. The most common reason for neck and shoulder problems results from the massage therapist using upper body _____ to exert the pressure for massage. Tense wrists and hands will also contribute to _____ problems. These problems can be avoided if the student learns to use _____, leans with the body weight to provide pressure, avoids _____ and the use of upper body strength, and maintains a _____ hand and wrist while giving a massage.

The massage professional will need to protect his or her wrists by avoiding excessive _____ forces developed from delivery of massage methods. The massage therapist must learn to keep the lower back straight and avoid bending or curling at the _____ while working. An _____ stance, along with variations using a short and tall stool will also provide methods of protection. Knee problems can be avoided by honoring the basic stability design of the knee and frequently _____ the weight from foot to foot. The most efficient standing position involves the normal screw home or knee lock position in the last 15 degrees of _____. This position provides the _____ compressive force on the knee capsule, and the least muscular action for stability.

The human body is designed for movement and range of motion and not for the compressive forces required when giving a massage. Because of this, it is vital to use body _____ and not muscle strength to provide the pressure required during a massage. Massage primarily uses a force generated _____ and downward. Therefore, it is necessary to redistribute the center of gravity and the weight force by keeping the weight on the _____ leg and the _____ point at the object-contact point. The arm generating the pressure is _____ of the weight-bearing leg, which allows for proper counterbalance and prevents twisting of the body.

Attention to body mechanics begins _____ the massage is even started. The therapist's body should be _____ up with general aerobic activity and stretching. Throughout the massage day, _____ should be taken between each massage, and all of the muscles used to give a massage should be stretched. The massage table must be at a _____ height, which depends on the body size and style of the therapist. Should a mat on the floor be chosen for the work, the same principles will apply. The balance points will then be from the _____ instead of the feet. If the massage therapist can give a massage in a relaxed, efficient, and energy conserving manner, the client will be able to _____ and more easily accept the touch. Practice, practice, practice until body mechanics are _____ and efficient.

C. LABELING

Label the following figures with the correct phrases as offered below. Then place an X next to those figures that show correct body mechanics.

a. When using compressive force, the weight is kept on the back leg and foot and the client's body is directly in front of the practitioner.

b. Wrist at wrong angle with excessive compressive force on wrist

c. Therapist is reaching for the stroke and the equilateral triangle is lost

d. Incorrect position for forearm with pressure against ulnar nerve

e. Knees in incorrect position with weight-bearing leg not stabilized in correct knee lock position

f. Pulling instead of leaning for stretch

g. For stretching, weight begins on front foot and shifts to back foot

h. Pulling tissue by lifting up

i. Pushing instead of lean for compressive force

j. Knees in hyperextension

k. Tight fingers instead of relaxed hand

l. Tight wrist and hand instead of relaxed wrist and hand

m. Weight on front foot for compressive forces and therapist is pushing instead of leaning for pressure. Wrist angle is wrong.

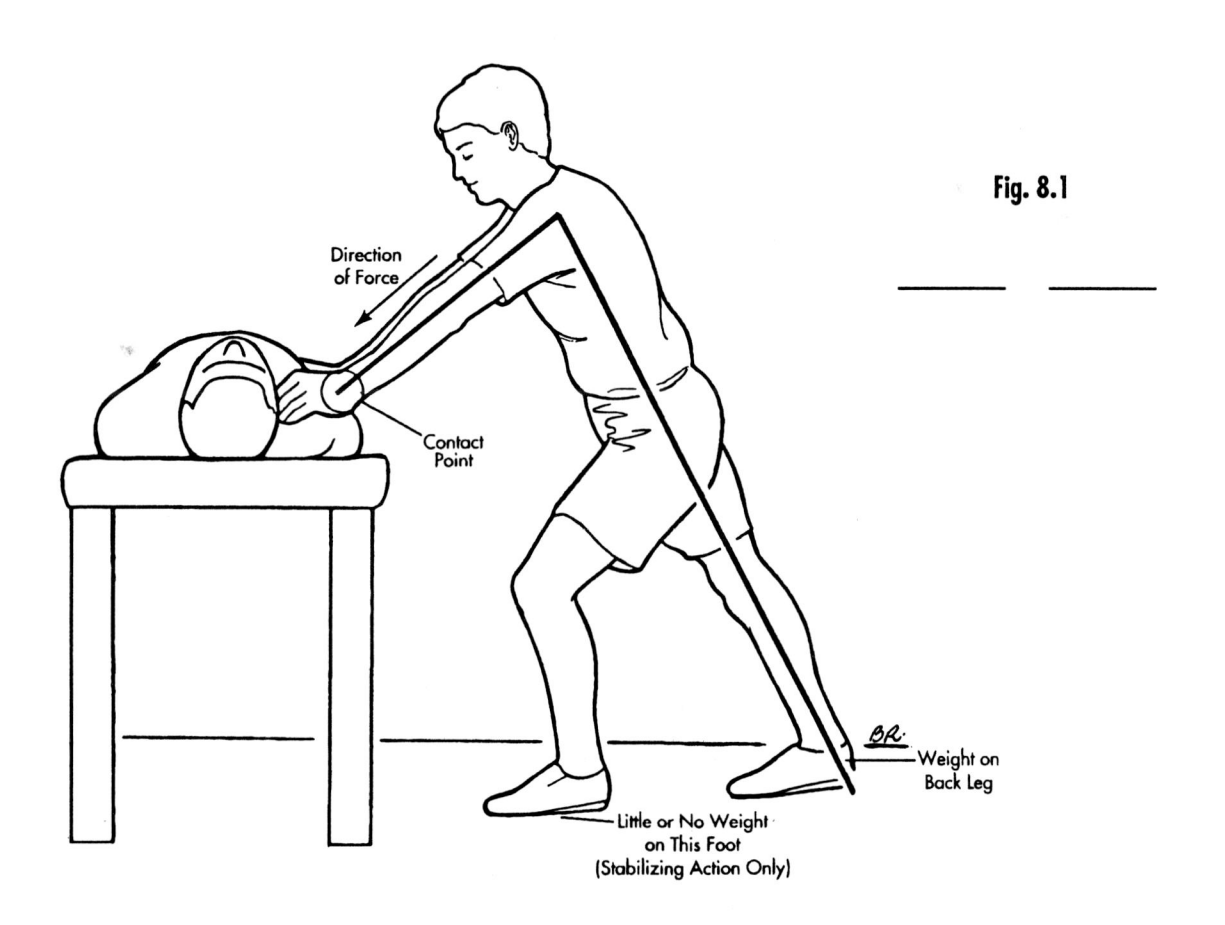

Fig. 8.1

_____ _____

C. LABELING (cont.)

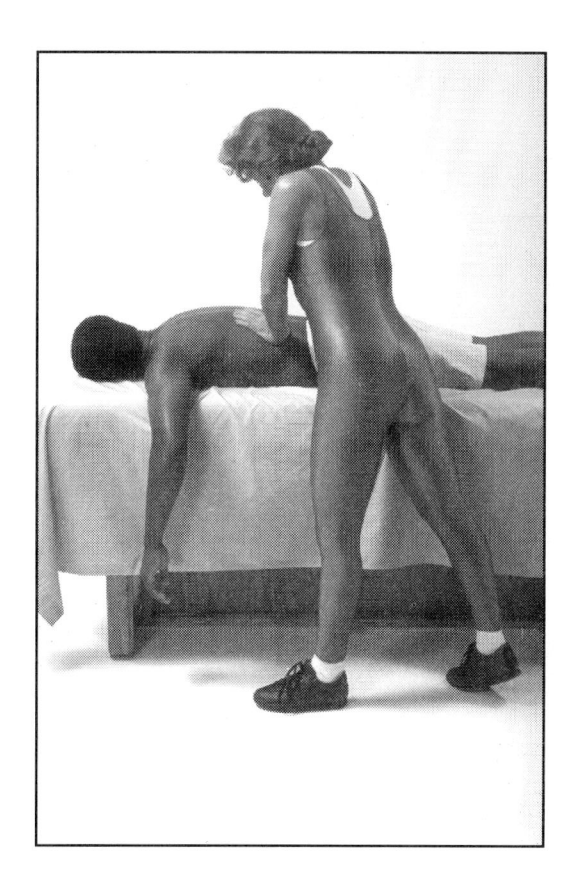

Fig. 8.2

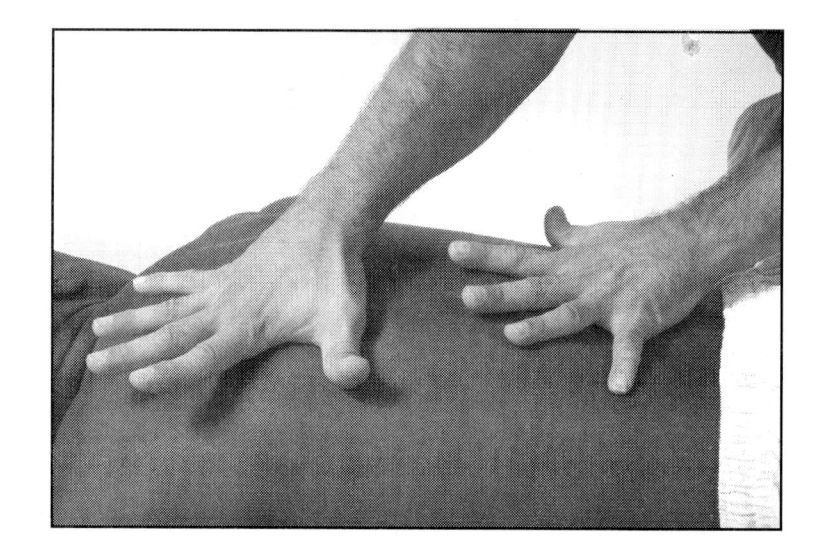

_____ _____

Fig. 8.3

_____ _____

C. LABELING (cont.)

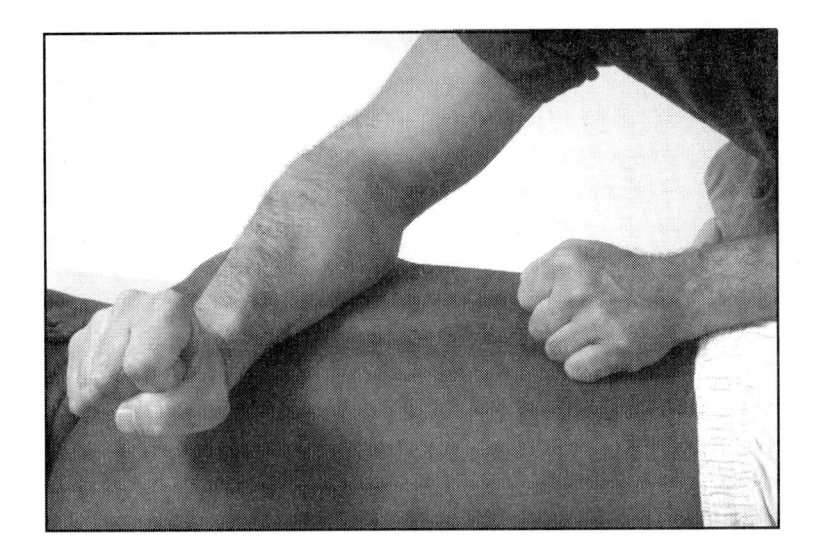

Fig. 8.4

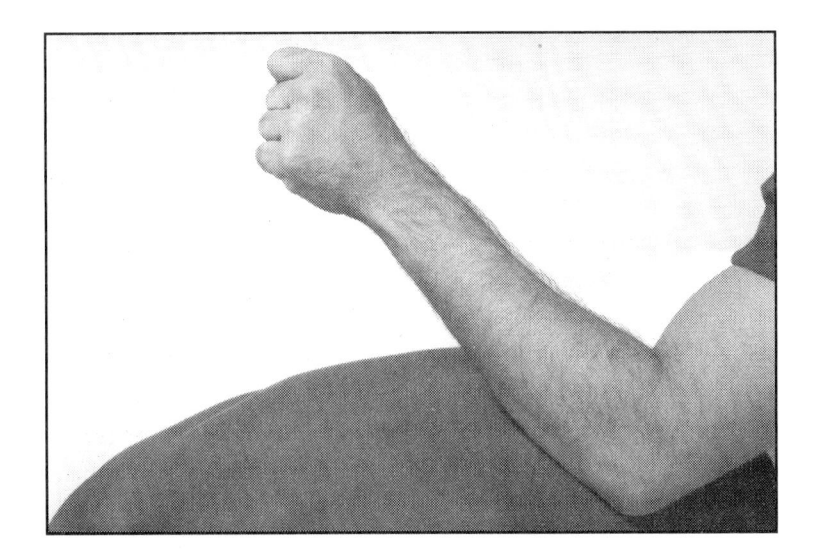

_____   _____

Fig. 8.5

_____   _____

C. LABELING (cont.)

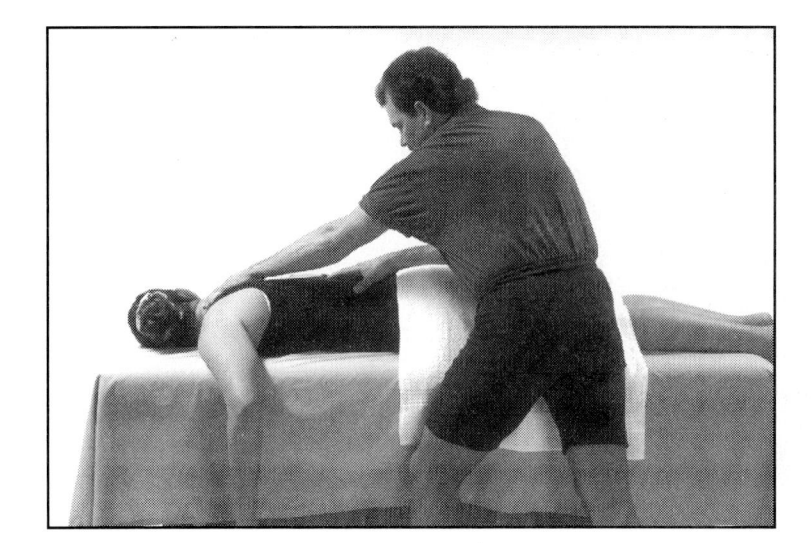

Fig. 8.6

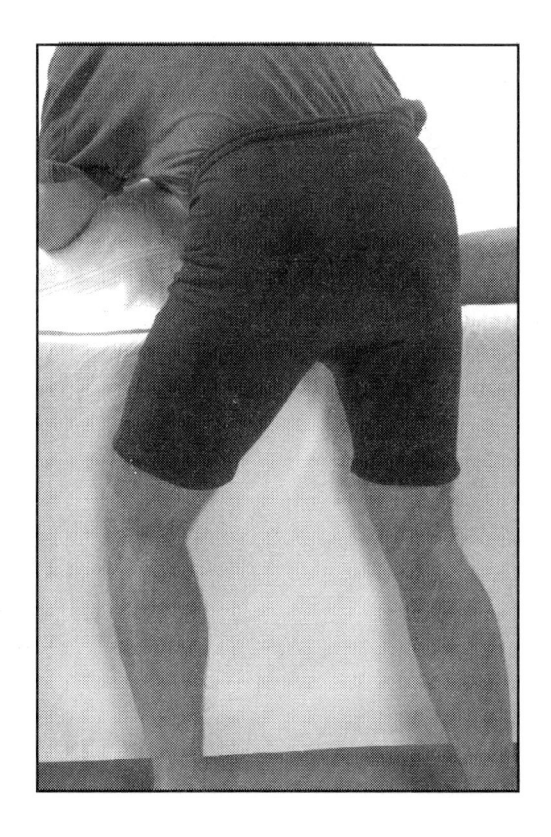

_____ _____

Fig. 8.7

_____ _____

Chapter 8

C. LABELING (cont.)

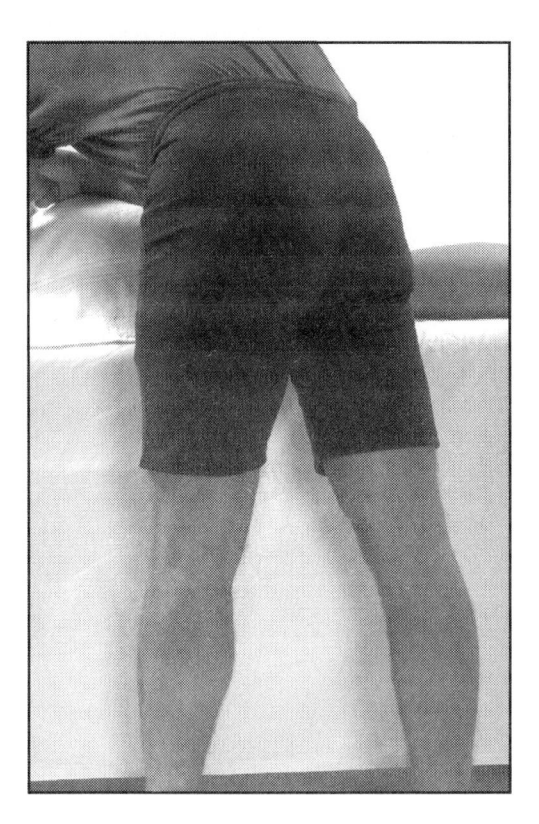

Fig. 8.8

_____ _____

Fig. 8.9

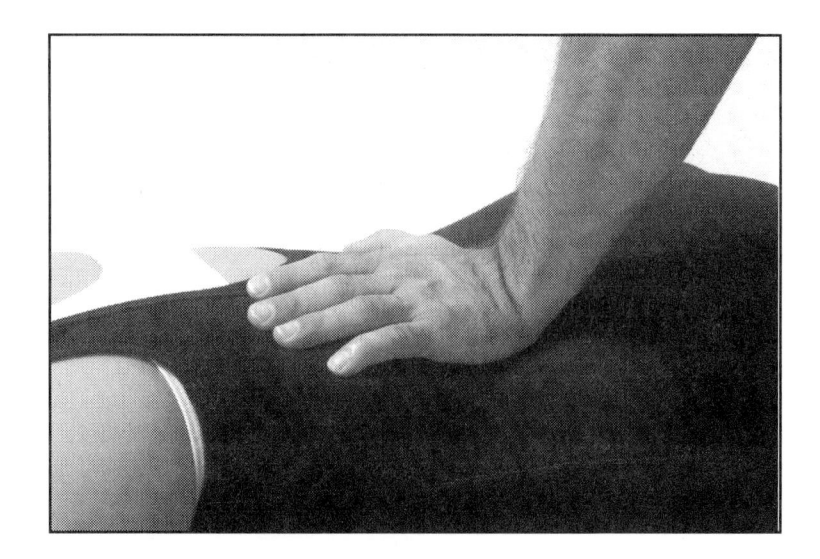

_____ _____

C. LABELING (cont.)

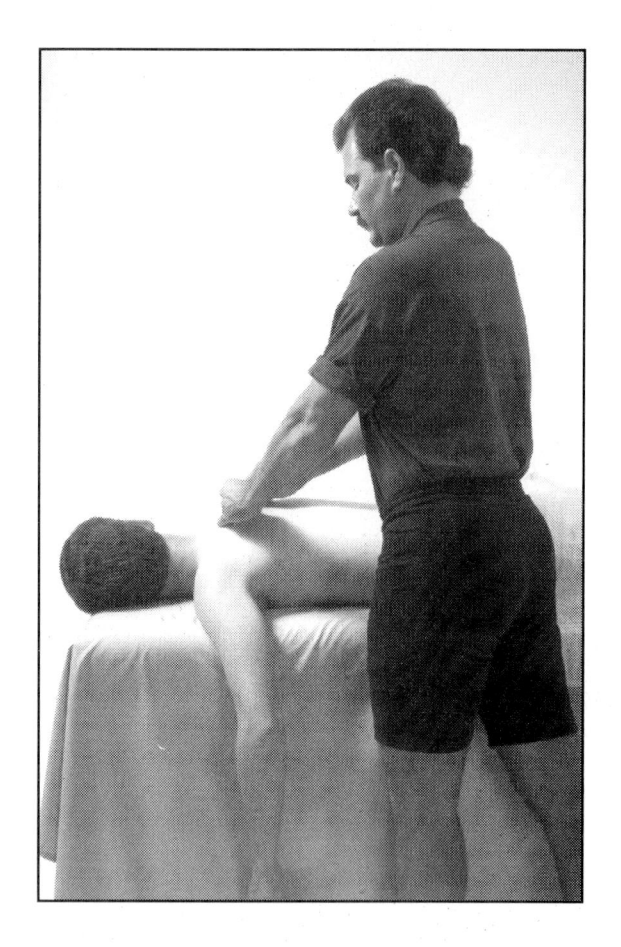

Fig. 8.10

_____   _____

Fig. 8.11

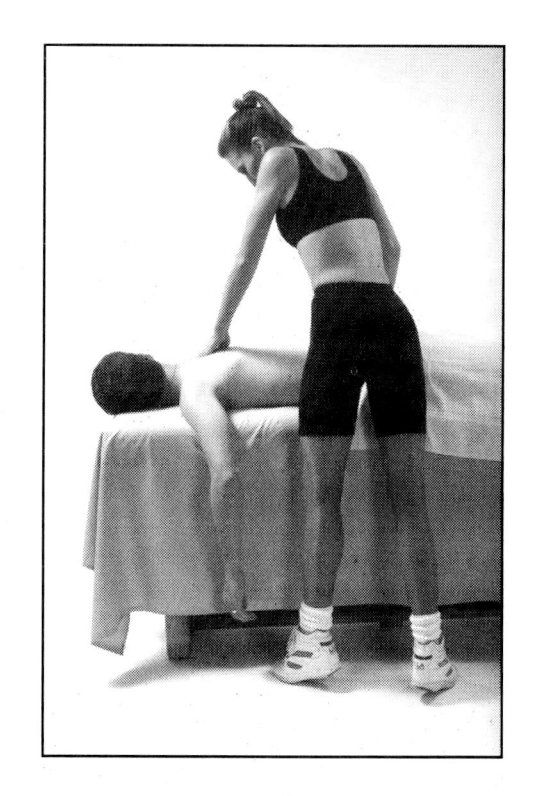

_____   _____

C. LABELING (cont.)

Fig. 8.12

_____   _____

"Lean Back"

Direction of Force

Weight Bearing Begins on Front Foot

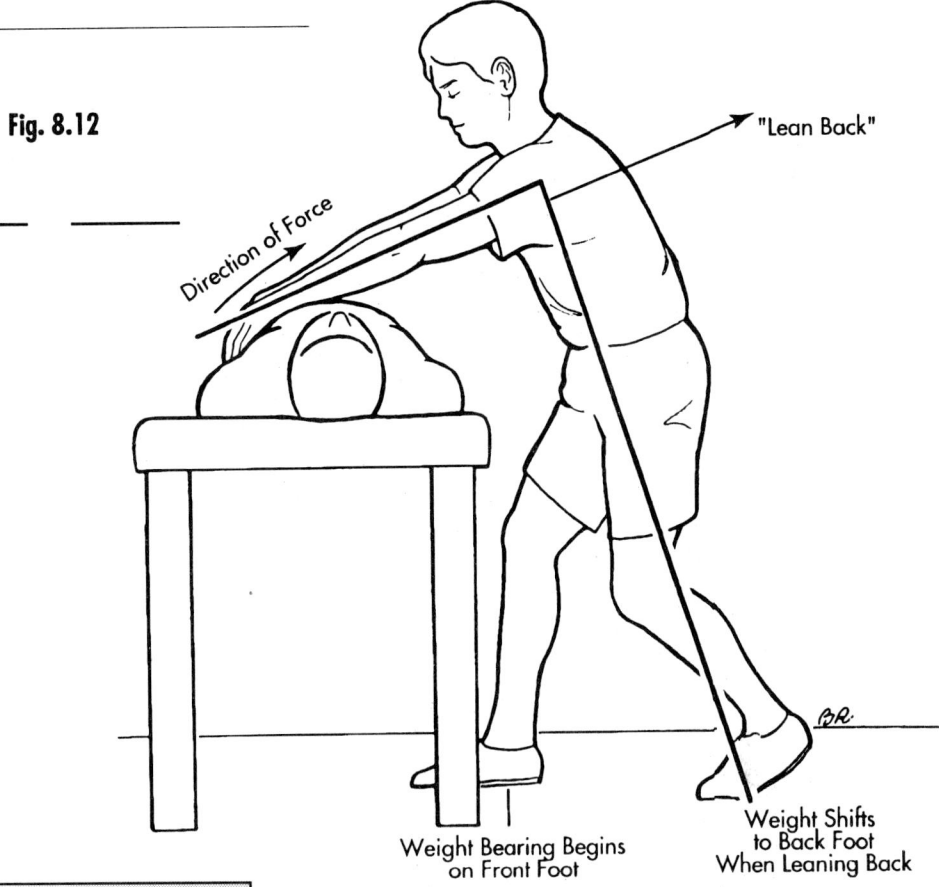

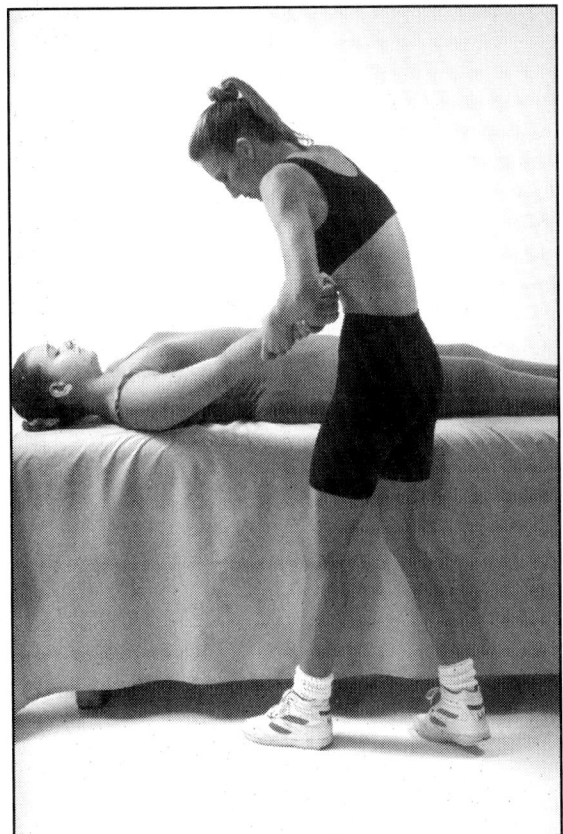

Weight Shifts to Back Foot When Leaning Back

Fig. 8.13

_____   _____

Body Mechanics

D. ADDITIONAL ACTIVITY

Cross out the incorrect word in the parenthesis found in each sentence. The finished result will reflect a true statement.

1. Areas of the body commonly affected in the massage professional who is not attentive to body mechanics (usually, do not) include the neck and shoulder, the wrist and thumb, low back, knee, ankle, and foot.

2. Some reasons for (wrist, low back) problems include inappropriate bending, bent static positions, twisting, and reaching while giving a massage.

3. Knee problems can be avoided by honoring the basic stability design of the knee and (frequently, avoiding) shifting the weight from foot to foot.

4. (Asymmetrical, symmetrical) standing with the weight equal on both feet is fatiguing, interferes with circulation, and should be avoided.

5. Massage (never, primarily) uses a force generated forward and downward.

6. The arm generating the pressure is (opposite, on the same side) of the weight-bearing leg, allowing for proper counterbalance and prevent twisting of the body.

7. Static and dynamic postures assumed at work and during recreational activities may have adverse effects on the body. These problems usually manifest in the (digestive, muscular skeletal) system.

8. Massage is physical work, but it is (less, more) like a dance or gymnastics than construction work.

9. Since the (client's body, therapist's hand) is the stabilizing point, we automatically mold ourselves to the client. The practitioner becomes extremely sensitive to subtle body changes in the client and bodywork takes on a dramatic new dimension.

10. Attention to body mechanics begins (once, before) the massage is started.

11. Besides getting a professional massage (weekly, monthly), the therapist should massage his or her own hands, arms, and shoulders during the day.

12. Should a mat on the floor be chosen for the work, the same principles will apply. The balance points will then be from the (hips, knees) instead of the feet.

13. Floor work is (very, not as) effective and the massage professional should be able to efficiently work from the floor.

14. The therapist's body must be in good alignment, with the feet in a (wide, narrow) base of support. The arm generating the downward pressure is opposite the back weight-bearing leg.

15. It is important to stay (behind, on top of) the stroke.

ANSWERS

1. KEY TERMS

1. d
2. a
3. b
4. c

B. FILL IN THE BLANKS

Body mechanics
burnout
posture
strength
shoulder
leverage
pushing
relaxed

compressive
waist
asymmetrical
shifting
extension
least

weight
forward
back
balance
opposite

before
warmed
breaks
comfortable
knees
relax
graceful

C. LABELING

1. a X
2. m
3. k
4. l
5. d
6. c
7. e
8. j
9. b
10. h
11. i
12. g X
13. f

D. ADDITIONAL ACTIVITY

These are the words which should be included in the statements.

1. usually
2. low back
3. frequently
4. Symmetrical
5. primarily
6. opposite
7. muscular skeletal
8. more
9. client's body
10. before
11. weekly
12. knees
13. very
14. wide
15. behind

CHAPTER 9

Getting Ready to Touch

A. KEY TERMS

Match the term to the best definition.

1. amenities _____
2. body supports _____
3. client expectations _____
4. client information form _____
5. client outcome _____
6. cream _____
7. drape _____
8. draping _____
9. history _____
10. lubricant _____
11. massage chair _____
12. massage environment _____
13. massage equipment _____
14. massage mat _____
15. massage procedures _____
16. massage table _____
17. oil _____
18. powder _____
19. pre-massage activities _____
20. wellness personal service _____

a. Document used to obtain information from the client about health, pre-existing conditions, and expectations of the massage.
b. The desired results from the massage and the massage therapist.
c. Additional items, such as music, that add to the comfort of the client.
d. Type of lubricant that is in a semi-solid or solid state.
e. Fabric used to cover the client and keep the client warm while the massage is given.
f. Specially designed piece of equipment that allows for a comfortable seated position during massage.
g. Area and location that massage is given.
h. Activities to prepare the client for the massage such as taking a client history, explaining how to get on the massage table, how drapes are used.

i. Specially designed equipment that allows massage to be done with the client lying down.

j. Type of liquid lubricant.

k. The procedures of covering and uncovering areas of the body and turning the client during the massage.

l. Ideas and expected results of the client based on past experience with massage, or from outside information.

m. Information from the client about past and present medical conditions, and patterns of symptoms.

n. Substance that reduces friction on the skin during massage movements.

o. Massage tables, mats, chairs, and other incidental supplies and implements used during massage.

p. Cushion that is used for floor work.

q. Massage that is used for general health enhancement and is not focused toward any specific medical condition.

r. Pillows, folded blankets, specially designed foam, or commercial products that help contour the flat surface of a massage table or mat.

s. Any activity that is involved in preparation for a massage including set up of the massage room, obtaining supplies, determining temperature of the room.

t. Type of lubricant that consists of a finely ground substance.

B. FILL IN THE BLANKS

All massage tables need to be checked _____ for structural stability. It is important to do a complete _____ on all the connectors, bolts, cables, and hinges every week, and repair any defects immediately. _____ are used to bolster the body during the massage and to provide _____ to the flat working surface. The purpose of using an _____ draping material is to provide the client with privacy and warmth. Sheets made out of _____ are the best choice because they do not slip on the client. Because _____ are smaller, a client may feel more exposed and prefer the security offered by a sheet. The best recommendation is to use two _____, one for the bottom and one for the top. If working with someone who has sensitive skin, use _____ to reduce the risk of a reaction.

Cover all body supports and pillows with pillow cases. Anytime _____ come in contact with the client, they must be laundered in an approved fashion before being used again. _____ serve only one purpose for the massage practitioner: they reduce friction on the skin during gliding-type massage strokes. Lubricants are classified as _____, _____, and _____. All lubricants must be dispensed from a _____ container. Headaches and other allergic responses to a lubricant are often from the volatile oils of _____ products.

Conditions for massage areas that need to be considered are the room _____ and fresh air supply. It is suggested that the massage room be kept at _____. Massage produces a _____ effect, which brings the blood closer to the surface, and allows internal heat to escape, cooling the client.

Clients will require _____ for removal of clothing in preparation for massage treatment. It is necessary to designate a massage site separate from the _____ location. The business or reception area should be near the _____, but privacy must be provided when taking the client history. In addition to a massage table, draping material, and supports, it is desirable to have disposable tissues, a clock and _____ available. The best recommendation is for the massage therapist to choose a variety of music, and then offer this collection for the client to _____ from for the session. The music itself can be very helpful in _____ the massage. _____ work in a dark room or by candle light because an open flame is a safety hazard. Many clients are also environmentally sensitive and react to _____. Avoid heavy use of aftershave, perfume, _____ cosmetic products, or hair spray.

Clients seeking basic wellness personal service for health enhancement need to understand the _____ of this level of education. The massage practitioner needs to _____ the client so that the expectations of the effects of massage are for increased general well being and efficient body function. Once the client understands the scope of practice of massage, the type of massage that will be provided to fit with his or her expectations, and the general outcome for the massage has been determined, then it is time to take a_____. The reasons for a history are to determine _____, decide if the client needs to be referred, and provide information for designing the massage.

While waiting for the client to prepare for the massage, it is important for the therapist to do the same. The goal is to be _____ in the moment for the client and not focused on lists of things that need to be done.

After the client is dressed and ready to leave, make the next appointment or provide a reminder if it already has been made. In some situations, a quick friendly _____ is appropriate only if initiated by the client.

C. PUZZLE

Find the following words in the word search.

amenities
client expectations
cream
drape
draping
environment
history
location
lubricant
massage chair
massage mat
oil
powder
set up
supplies
wellness

```
D H A B Z Y X W V U T N E M N O R I V N E
R J T S E I T I N E M A A P P H O M Y B N
A L S M A S S A G E C H A I R M G K M D V
P N A A G G C U Y L F T C S E A Q P C F W
I P Q T D N Z R I D G D E A D S C U A E R
N R Y N L I O N E G Z T R F W S O V L H N
G T O A V T I Q P A I E G A O A N L O J O
F V L C S T L P U O M L I D P G N W C L M
E X L I T C J O T B Y W K B E E T X A N E
D Z H R A E R S E I L P P U S M U Y T P N
C N E B C P T W S T D E M S A A S Z I Q T
B O S U E X M U S L E C O L R T W G O R A
A T C L I E N T E X P E C T A T I O N S B
```

D. MATCHING

1. Fill in the blanks in the sentence with the correct terms from the list given. There is one correct answer for each statement, but not all of the terms will be used.

To help a person off of the table:

1. Reach under the client's ____.
2. Support the sheet loosely around the client's neck and hold it so that it does not slip ____.
3. Lift the client's torso off the table while swinging the knees around ____.
4. Stabilize the client for a moment ____.
5. Still holding the sheet, ____.
6. Shift the position of the sheet so that the client ____.

If a client is left to get off the table alone, the following reminders should be given to the client.

7. Roll to ____.
8. Use the arms to push ____.
9. Sit for a minute ____.
10. Leave the sheets ____.
11. Get dressed and ____.

a. nose
b. neck and knees
c. when the music stops
d. and around
e. then spin again
f. when the person is lifted
g. in case of dizziness
h. to a seated position
i. cannot see the therapist
j. the floor

k. return to the business area
l. the client away
m. on the table
n. then go away
o. can hold it securely
p. help the client to a standing position
q. one side
r. to the edge of the table
s. before getting up

2. *Match the statement with the correct massage equipment it describes:*

A - PORTABLE MASSAGE TABLE
B - MASSAGE CHAIR
C - MASSAGE MAT

Place the correct letter next to the following statements.

1. Sturdy construction using cable support on the legs. _____
2. Large enough for the massage practitioner to move around the client's body while staying on the cushioned surface to protect the knees and body. _____
3. Professionally manufactured, lightweight and portable, providing comfortable seated massage. _____
4. Safety: there is little chance of a client falling. _____
5. A face cradle. _____
6. Manual height adjustment. _____
7. Some people have difficulty getting in and out of the semi-kneeling position. _____
8. A popular choice when working with infants and children _____
9. Proper training needed to work effectively on the floor _____
10. It should be 30 inches wide (most are about six feet long). Less that 30 inches wide is too narrow for client comfort. If wider, it becomes difficult to carry _____

E. ADDITIONAL ACTIVITY

Determine which of the following statements are false. For those items that are false, write false on the answer space provided.

1. Interview a client to better understand the clients's expectations of massage in general and the outcome for a massage session in particular. _____
2. Obtain a history from the client for the purposes of identifying contraindications. _____
3. Obtain a history from the client for the purposes of determining the need for referral. _____
4. Obtain a history from the client for the purposes of determining a diagnosis of a specific condition. _____
5. Obtain informed consent from the client before the massage session begins. _____
6. Take client to the massage area. _____
7. Show the client where clothes may be hung. _____
8. Instruct client that he or she must remove all clothing. _____
9. Instruct client to remove amount of clothing he or she is comfortable with and leave on underclothing for additional comfort or security. _____
10. Show how the draping will work. _____

11. If using a massage chair or other set up, show the client how to use it for proper positioning. _____
12. Point out the rest room location and the procedure for getting there if it is not located next to the massage area. _____
13. Do not offer a choice of the type of lubricant or have the option for no lubricant. _____
14. Remain in the room with all clients as they disrobe to prepare for the massage. _____
15. Explain all sanitary precautions and show these to the client. _____
16. Lock the door to the massage room. _____
17. Give a general idea of the massage flow. _____
18. If there is any chance that the client may fall or need assistance getting on or off the table, stay in the room to help. _____
19. Do not announce yourself before entering the massage room. _____

F. PROBLEM SOLVING EXERCISES

1. A client indicates on the client information form that he does not wish to have an oil-based lubricant used on his back, face, or chest. What are your options?

   _____
   _____
   _____
   _____

2. You are scheduled to travel to a client's home to do a massage. When you arrive you realize that there is no private location large enough to accommodate the massage table. What are some of your options?

   _____
   _____
   _____
   _____

G. PROFESSIONAL APPLICATION

You have been contracted to provide on-site massage in an office setting using a chair. Before you begin, you will have a chance to visit the location. List the specifics you will look for in locating the massage area, what supplies you need to include in the traveling office, and what materials you will need.

_____
_____
_____
_____

H. RESEARCH FOR FURTHER STUDY

Access various nursing texts and study positioning and draping procedures; record any procedures that are applicable to massage.

ANSWERS

A. KEY TERMS

1. c
2. r
3. l
4. a
5. b
6. d
7. e
8. k
9. m
10. n
11. f
12. g
13. o
14. p
15. h
16. i
17. j
18. t
19. s
20. q

B. FILL IN THE BLANKS

daily
maintenance check
Body supports
contour
opaque
cotton
towels
twin size flat cotton sheets
white pure cotton sheets

linens
Lubricants
oils
creams
powders
contamination free
scented

temperature
75°
vasodilation

privacy
business
entrance
music
choose
pacing
Never
scents
scented

limitations
educate
history
contraindications

present

hug

C. PUZZLE

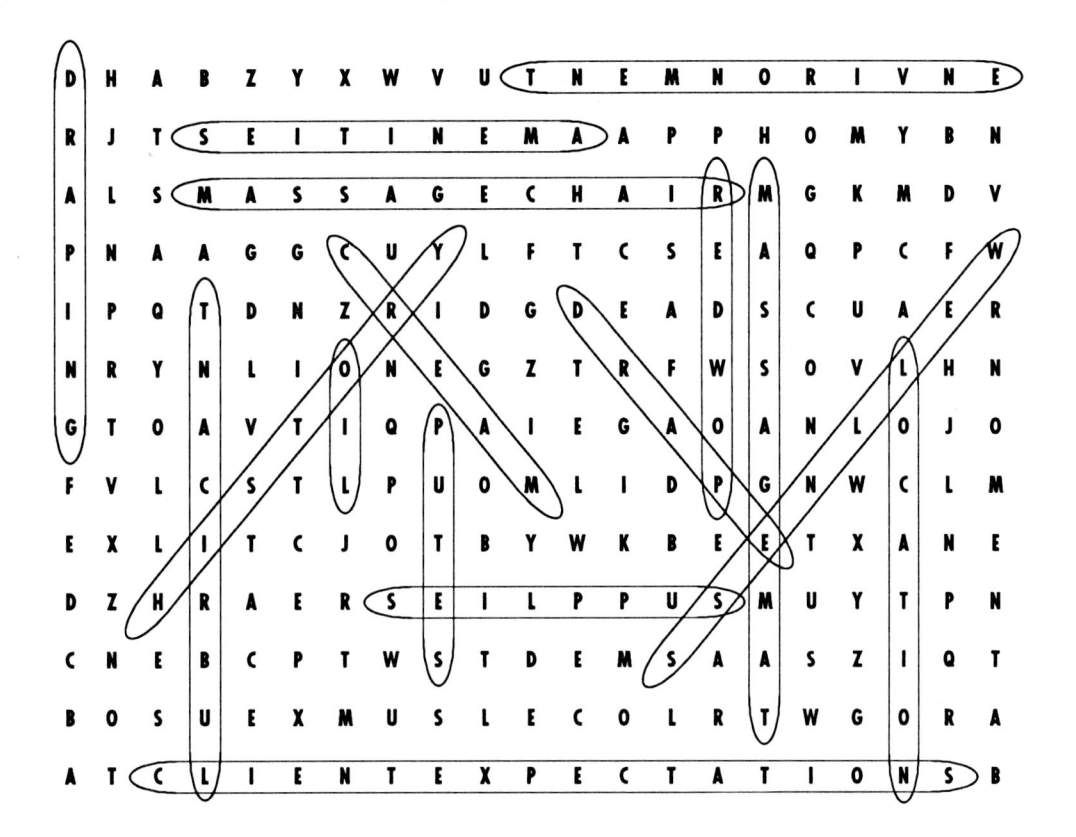

D	H	A	B	Z	Y	X	W	V	U	T	N	E	M	N	O	R	I	V	N	E
R	J	T	S	E	I	T	I	N	E	M	A	A	P	P	H	O	M	Y	B	N
A	L	S	M	A	S	S	A	G	E	C	H	A	I	R	M	G	K	M	D	V
P	N	A	A	G	G	C	U	Y	L	F	T	C	S	E	A	Q	P	C	F	W
I	P	Q	T	D	N	Z	R	I	D	G	D	E	A	D	S	C	U	A	E	R
N	R	Y	N	L	I	O	N	E	G	Z	T	R	F	W	S	O	V	L	H	N
G	T	O	A	V	T	I	Q	P	A	I	E	G	A	O	A	N	L	O	J	O
F	V	L	C	S	T	L	P	U	O	M	L	I	D	P	G	N	W	C	L	M
E	X	L	I	T	C	J	O	T	B	Y	W	K	B	E	E	T	X	A	N	E
D	Z	H	R	A	E	R	S	E	I	L	P	P	U	S	M	U	Y	T	P	N
C	N	E	B	C	P	T	W	S	T	D	E	M	S	A	A	S	Z	I	Q	T
B	O	S	U	E	X	M	U	S	L	E	C	O	L	R	T	W	G	O	R	A
A	T	C	L	I	E	N	T	E	X	P	E	C	T	A	T	I	O	N	S	B

D. MATCHING

1.
   1. b
   2. f
   3. r
   4. g
   5. p
   6. o
   7. q
   8. h
   9. s
   10. m
   11. k

2.
   1. A
   2. C
   3. B
   4. C
   5. A or B
   6. A
   7. B
   8. C
   9. C
   10. A

E. ADDITIONAL ACTIVITY

The following items are false: 4, 8, 13, 14, 16, 19

F. PROBLEM SOLVING EXERCISES

1. Use of powder or water-based cream. Compression-type massage over a clean sheet or towel in these areas.
2. Switch to an over-the-clothing massage and request that the client change into loose, non-restrictive clothing. Turn the session into an educational session teaching others in the household to do some simple massage techniques. Do a seated massage in a private location.

CHAPTER 10

Massage Manipulations and Techniques

A. KEY TERMS

Match the term to the best definition.

1. Match the massage manipulation or technique with its description.

1. active joint movement _____
2. beating _____
3. compression _____
4. cross-directional stretching _____
5. cupping _____
6. effleurage (gliding stroke) _____
7. friction _____
8. hacking _____
9. joint movement _____
10. lengthening _____
11. longitudinal stretching _____
12. manipulation _____
13. muscle energy techniques _____
14. passive joint movement _____
15. petrissage (kneading) _____
16. positional release _____
17. post isometric relaxation _____
18. proprioceptive neuromuscular facilitation (PNF) _____
19. pulsed muscle energy _____
20. reciprocal inhibition (RI) _____
21. resting stroke _____
22. rocking _____
23. shaking _____
24. skin-rolling _____
25. slapping _____
26. stretching _____
27. stroke _____
28. tapotement _____
29. tapping _____
30. techniques _____
31. traction _____
32. vibration _____

a. Type of alternating tapotement that strikes the surface of the body with quick snapping movements.

b. The movement of the joint through its normal range-of-motion.

c. The assuming of a normal resting length by a muscle through the neuromuscular mechanism.

d. A stretch applied along the fiber direction of the connective tissues and muscles.

e. Tissue stretching that pulls and twists connective tissue against its fiber direction.

f. By moving the body out of the position causing discomfort and into the direction it wants to go, the proprioception is taken into a state of safety and may stop signalling for protective spasm.

g. Occurs after an isometric contraction of a muscle, resulting from the activity of minute neural reporting stations called the Golgi tendon bodies.

h. Application of muscle energy techniques that combines muscle contractions with stretching and muscular pattern retraining.

i. Rhythmical movement of the body.

j. Body area is grasped and shaken in a quick loose movement. Sometimes classified as rhythmic mobilization.

k. A form of petrissage that lifts skin.

l. The client produces the movement of a joint through its range of movement.

m. Methods of therapeutic massage that provide sensory stimulation or mechanical alteration of the soft tissue of the body.

n. Pressure into the body to spread tissue against underlying structures. This massage manipulation is sometimes classified with petrissage.

o. Gentle pull on the joint capsule to increase the joint space.

p. Fine or coarse tremulous movement that creates reflexive responses.

q. A type of tapotement that uses a cupped hand often used over the thorax.

r. Horizontal strokes applied with the fingers, hand, or forearm that usually follow the fiber direction of the underlying muscle, fascial planes, or a dermatome pattern.

s. Specific circular or transverse movements that are focused to the underlying tissue and do not glide on the skin.

t. Procedures that involve engaging the barrier and using minute, resisted, contractions (usually 20 in 10 seconds) which introduces mechanical pumping as well as PIR or RI (depending on the muscles used).

u. Takes place when a muscle contracts, obliging its antagonist to relax in order to allow normal movement to take place.

v. First stroke of the massage. The simple laying on of hands.

w. Form of tapotement that uses a flat hand.

x. Mechanical tension applied to lengthen the myofascial unit (muscles and fascia). Two types exist: longitudinal and cross-directional.

y. A form of heavy tapotement that uses the fist.

z. A technique of therapeutic massage that is applied with a movement on the surface of the body whether superficial or deep.

aa. Springy blows to the body at a fast rate to create rhythmical compression to the tissue. Also called percussion.

bb. Type of tapotement done using the finger tips.

cc. Skillful use of the hands in a therapeutic manner. Massage manipulations are focused to the soft tissues of the body and are not to be confused with joint manipulation using a high velocity thrust.

dd. Specific use of active contraction in individual or groups of muscles to initiate a relaxation response. Activation of the proprioceptors to facilitate muscle tone, relaxation, and stretching.

ee. The massage practitioner moves the jointed areas without the assistance of the client.

ff. Rhythmic rolling, lifting, squeezing, and wringing of soft tissue.

2. *Match the movement activity with its proper description.*

1. arthrokinematic movement _____
2. concentric isotonic contraction _____
3. counterpressure _____
4. eccentric isotonic contraction _____
5. isokinetic contraction _____
6. isometric contraction _____
7. isotonic contraction _____
8. osteokinematic movements _____

a. Accessory movements that occur because of inherent laxity or joint play that exists in each joint. These essential movements occur passively with movement of the joint, and are not under voluntary control.

b. During the contraction of a muscle, the massage therapist applies a counterforce but allows the client to move, bringing origin and insertion of the target muscle together against the pressure.

c. The effort of the target muscle, or group of muscles, is greater than the counterpressure, allowing a degree of resisted movement to occur.

d. Flexion, extension, abduction, adduction, and rotation. Also referred to as physiologic movements.

e. Contraction in which the effort of the muscle, or group of muscles, is exactly matched by a counterpressure, so that no movement occurs, only effort.

f. The client moves the joint through a full range of motion, using full muscle strength, against partial resistance supplied by the massage therapist. This is therefore a multiple isotonic movement.

g. During the extension of a muscle, the massage therapist applies a counterforce but allows the client to move the jointed area to let origin and insertion separate.

h. The force produced by the muscles of a specific area which is designed to match the effort exactly (isometric contraction) or partially (isotonic contraction).

3. Match the term with the proper definition.

1. antagonists _____
2. barrier _____
3. compressive force _____
4. depth of pressure _____
5. direction _____
6. direction of ease _____
7. drag _____
8. facilitation _____
9. Golgi tendon receptors _____
10. heavy pressure _____
11. inhibition _____
12. insertion _____
13. joint kinesthetic receptors _____
14. moderate pressure _____
15. motor point _____
16. neuromuscular mechanism _____
17. origin _____
18. positioning _____
19. pressure _____
20. prime movers _____
21. proprioceptors _____
22. range-of-motion _____
23. refractory period _____
24. reflex _____
25. soft tissue _____
26. spindle cells _____
27. stabilization _____
28. stimulation _____
29. superficial fascia _____
30. superficial pressure _____
31. target muscles _____
32. tone _____
33. tonic vibration reflex _____
34. touch _____

a. A limitation in movement. Anatomic barriers are caused by the fit of the bones at the joint. Physiologic barriers are from the limits of range-of-motion from protective nerve and sensory function.

b. Contact with no movement.

c. Some sort of excitation that activate the sensory nerves.

d. Connective tissue layer just under the skin.

e. A compressive stress that can be light, moderate, deep, and variable.

f. Pressure that stays on the skin.

g. The muscle or groups of muscles that the response of the methods is specifically focused upon.

h. State of causing the muscle to contract or strengthen.

i. Reflex that tones a muscle with stimulation through vibration methods at the tendon.

j. The amount of pull on the tissue.

k. The muscles that oppose the movement of the prime movers.

l. The state of a nerve when it is stimulated, but not to the point of threshold where it will transmit a nerve signal.

m. The body assumes postural changes and muscle shortening or weakening depending upon how it has balanced against gravity.

n. Flow of massage strokes can be from the center of the body out (centrifugal), or from the extremities in toward the center of the body (centripetal). It can be from origin to insertion of the muscle following the muscle fibers, transverse to the tissue fibers, or in a circular motion.

o. Compressive pressure that extend to the muscle layer but does not press the tissue against the underlying bone.
p. Placing the body in such a way that specific joints of muscles are isolated.
q. Compressive force.
r. Amount of pressure against the surface of the body to apply pressure to the deeper body structures.
s. The muscles responsible for a movement.
t. One of three types of sensory nerves in the joint that detect position and speed of movement.
u. Point at which a motor nerve enters the muscle it innervates and will cause a muscle twitch if stimulated.
v. Movement of joints.
w. Response that is dependent on nervous system function. Reflexive methods work by causing a stimulation of the nervous system (sensory neurons) and the tissue changes in response to the body's adaptation to the neural stimulation.
x. Holding the body in a fixed position during joint movement, lengthening, and stretching.
y. Sensory receptors in the belly of the muscle that detect stretch.
z. The skin, fascia, muscles, tendons, joint capsules, and ligaments of the body.
aa. Amount of time that a muscle will be unable to contract after it has contracted.
bb. Sensory receptors that detect joint and muscle activity.
cc. Attachment point of a muscle at the fixed point during movement.
dd. The interplay and reflex connection between sensory and motor neurons and muscle function.
ee. Receptors in the tendons that sense tension.
ff. Compressive force that extends to the bone under the tissue.
gg. To decrease or cease a response or function.
hh. The muscle attachment point that is closest to the moving joint.

B. FILL IN THE BLANKS

In general, massage methods and techniques stimulate or _____ response.

The act of placing your hand on another person seems so simple, yet this initial contact must be made with _____ and a client-centered focus. With this technique, we enter the client's personal _____ space, defined by sensitivity to changes in air pressure and movement picked up by the sensory receptors in the _____. It gives the client time to evaluate, on a subconscious level, whether this touch is _____.

The current term for _____ is "gliding stroke." The most superficial applications of this stroke do this, but the full spectrum of effleurage is determined by pressure, drag, speed, direction, and rhythm, making this manipulation one of the most _____. The distinguishing characteristic of effleurage is that it is applied _____ in relation to the tissues.

Petrissage requires that the soft tissue be _____, rolled, and squeezed by the massage therapist. Just as effleurage is focused horizontally on the body, petrissage functions _____. Petrissage is very good for _____ in muscle tone. The lifting, rolling, and squeezing action affects the _____ proprioceptors in the muscle belly. When lifting, the _____ are stretched, thus increasing tension in both the tendons and the Golgi tendon receptors, which have a protective function.

_____ has developed as a distinct manipulation in recent years with the advents of sports massage and on-site corporate massage.

This manipulation is a way of working over the clothing or without _____. Very specific pinpoint compression is called direct pressure, or _____ compression, and is used on acupressure points (motor points) and trigger points. It is also very good to use on bodies that are _____ since the manipulations do not glide on the skin, pull the tissue, or require lubricant.

Manual vibration can be used successfully by the massage therapist to tone muscles by applying the technique at the muscle _____ for up to 30 seconds. Shaking manipulations confuse the _____ proprioceptors so the muscles relax. Shaking warms and prepares the body for deeper bodywork and works with joints in a _____ manner. _____ is a soothing and rhythmic form of shaking that has been used since the beginning of time to calm people. Rocking works though the vestibular system of the inner ear and feeds sensory input directly into the _____. For rocking to be most effective, the body must move so that the fluid in the semi-circular canals of the _____ are affected, initiating parasympathetic mechanisms.

Rocking is one of the most effective _____ techniques of the massage therapist. Many _____ responses are caused by the rocking of the body during the effleurage, petrissage, and compression methods.

Tapotement techniques require that the hands or parts of the hand administer springy _____ to the body at a fast rate. Tapotement is divided into two classifications, _____ and heavy. The strongest effect of tapotement is due to the response of the _____ reflexes. A quick blow to the tendon _____ it. In response, a protective muscle _____ results.

One method of _____ consists of small deep movements performed on a local area. The result of this type of friction is the initiation of a small controlled _____ response. Due to its specific nature and direct focus to rehabilitation, it is not suitable for the _____-level massage practitioner. A modified application of friction, used to keep areas of high concentration of connective tissue soft and pliable, is _____ for the beginner.

The efficient use of massage _____ will reduce the need for repetitive massage manipulations. If used well, the neuromuscular mechanism can be activated and influenced quickly with less _____ effort by the massage therapist.

The techniques of passive and active joint movement, muscle energy and proprioceptive neuromuscular facilitation techniques work with the neuromuscular reflex system to relax and _____ muscles. Stretching has both a reflexive and _____ effect and is more focused on the _____ tissue.

During a massage session, strive to move every joint approximately three times to gently encourage an increase in the _____. Proprioceptive neuromuscular facilitation (PNF) techniques developed out of physical therapy during the 1950s. It uses maximal contraction and rotary diagonal movement patterns to reeducate the _____ system. In recent years, the massage profession began to use pieces of the system to enhance _____, primarily in athletes. The diagonal movement patterns incorporate cross-body movement used in repatterning for children born with various forms of damage to the _____ areas of the brain. These types of movements reflexively stimulate the _____ or walking pattern and are a valuable addition to any massage system.

Muscle energy techniques involve a voluntary contraction of the client's muscle in a specific and controlled direction, at varying levels of intensity, against a specific _____ applied by the massage practitioner. Muscle energy procedures have a variety of applications and are considered _____ techniques in which the client contributes the corrective force. The amount of effort may vary from a _____ muscle twitch to a maximal muscle contraction. The _____ may last from a fraction of a second to several seconds. The focus of muscle energy techniques is to stimulate the nervous system to allow a more normal _____ length in muscles. To describe what happens, the proper term lengthening is used because _____ is more of a neurological response that allows the muscles to stop contracting and relax. _____ is a mechanical force applied to the tissue. Muscle energy techniques are focused to specific muscles or muscle groups. It is important to be able to _____ muscles so that the origin and insertion are either close together or in a lengthening phase with the origin and insertion _____.

Counterpressure is the force applied to an area that is designed to match the effort or force exactly _____ or partially _____. The response of the method is specific to a certain muscle or muscle groups referred to as the _____.

There are instances when the client does not or cannot participate actively in the massage. The principles of muscle energy techniques can still be used by _____ manipulation of the spindle cells or Golgi tendons.

Strain-counterstrain was formalized by Dr. Lawrence Jones and involves using _____ to guide the positioning of the body into a space where the muscle tension can release on its own. The tender points are often located in the _____ of the tight muscle due to the diagonal balancing process the body uses to maintain an upright posture against gravity. Positional release is a more _____ method that allows the beginning therapist to do similar work.

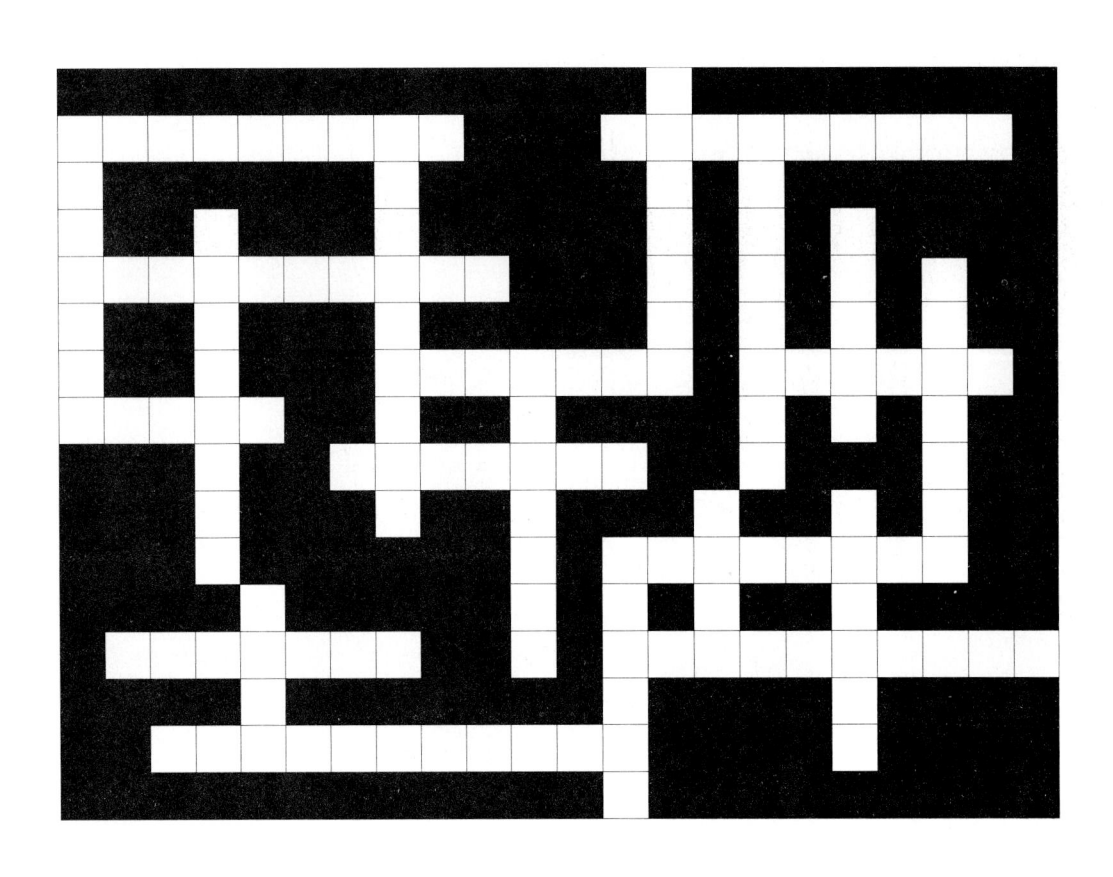

C. PUZZLE

Complete the puzzle by filling in the spaces with the following words.

transverse
rhythmic
reflexive
tapping
pliable
prone
rocking
supine
hacking
petrissage
vibration
resting

compression
cupping
lubricant
kneading
glide
shaking
manual
tissue
soothing
soft
skim

Chapter 10

D. MATCHING

Moving and Grooving with Massage: Match the phrase with the manipulation listed.

1. Jerry Lee Lewis does a whole lot of this. _____
2. The Beach Boys had a good one. _____
3. Your feet do this to the Electric Slide and the Hustle. _____
4. The two moves that make up the Mashed Potato. _____
5. The Buckingham's had kind of one. _____
6. You need to know this to stay in step with the other dancers. _____
7. The Swim. _____
8. Chubby Checker and the Twist. _____
9. This could keep you from dancing. _____
10. I've got this – do you? _____
11. This and roll(ing) is here to stay. _____
12. Music and muscle both have this. _____
13. How long has this been going on? _____
14. Fun dancing can be this. _____
15. What a tired waitress uses. _____
16. Younger brothers and sisters often try to be this. _____
17. The use of tissues. _____
18. The way some of us make our dough. _____
19. William Tell aimed for the apple, not this. _____
20. Putting coffee in containers. _____
21. Magnets have this for each other. _____

a. direction
b. inhibition
c. drag
d. rhythm
e. rocking
f. movement cure
g. cupping
h. target (muscle)
i. compression and friction
j. counterpressure
k. antagonists
l. cryotherapy
m. shaking
n. hydrotherapy
o. cross-directional stretching
p. tone
q. kneading
r. duration
s. gliding/effleurage
t. a traction
u. vibration

E. PROBLEM SOLVING EXERCISES

1. A client has tight muscles of the legs. She also has a history of varicose veins. The problem is not serious and there is no history of blood clots. This makes direct massage of the area contraindicated. What methods can be used to relax the legs?

2. A client has very sensitive skin and cannot have any type of lubricant used. What massage methods will you use.

3. A client's nose becomes stuffy; he gets a sinus headache when lying on his stomach. How will you give him a massage?

F. PROFESSIONAL APPLICATION

A massage therapist is finding that he is becoming fatigued with the style of massage he tends to provide, which consists mostly of effleurage, petrissage, and tapotement. He would like to be able to work more effectively. What recommendation can you provide?

ANSWERS

A. KEY TERMS

1.
   1. l
   2. y
   3. n
   4. e
   5. q
   6. r
   7. s
   8. a
   9. b
   10. c
   11. d
   12. cc
   13. dd
   14. ee
   15. ff
   16. f
   17. g
   18. h
   19. t
   20. u
   21. v
   22. i
   23. j
   24. k
   25. w
   26. x
   27. z
   28. aa
   29. bb
   30. m
   31. o
   32. p

2.
   1. a
   2. b
   3. h
   4. g
   5. f
   6. e
   7. c
   8. d

3.
   1. k
   2. a
   3. r
   4. e
   5. n
   6. m
   7. j
   8. l
   9. ee
   10. ff
   11. gg
   12. hh
   13. t
   14. o
   15. u
   16. dd
   17. cc
   18. p
   19. q
   20. s
   21. bb
   22. v
   23. aa
   24. w
   25. z
   26. y
   27. x
   28. c
   29. d
   30. f
   31. g
   32. h
   33. i
   34. b

B. FILL IN THE BLANKS

inhibit

respect
boundary
skin
safe

effleurage
versatile
horizontally

lifted
vertically
decreasing
spindle cell
tendons

Compression

lubricant
ischemic
hairy

tendons
positional
nonspecific
Rocking
cerebellum
inner ear

relaxation
parasympathetic

blows
light
tendon
stretches
contraction

friction
inflammatory
beginning
appropriate

techniques
physical

lengthen
mechanical
connective

range-of-motion
nervous
stretching
motor
gait

counterforce
active
small
duration
resting
Lengthening
Stretching
position
separated

(isometric contraction)
(isotonic contraction)
target muscle

direct

tender points
antagonist
general

C. PUZZLE

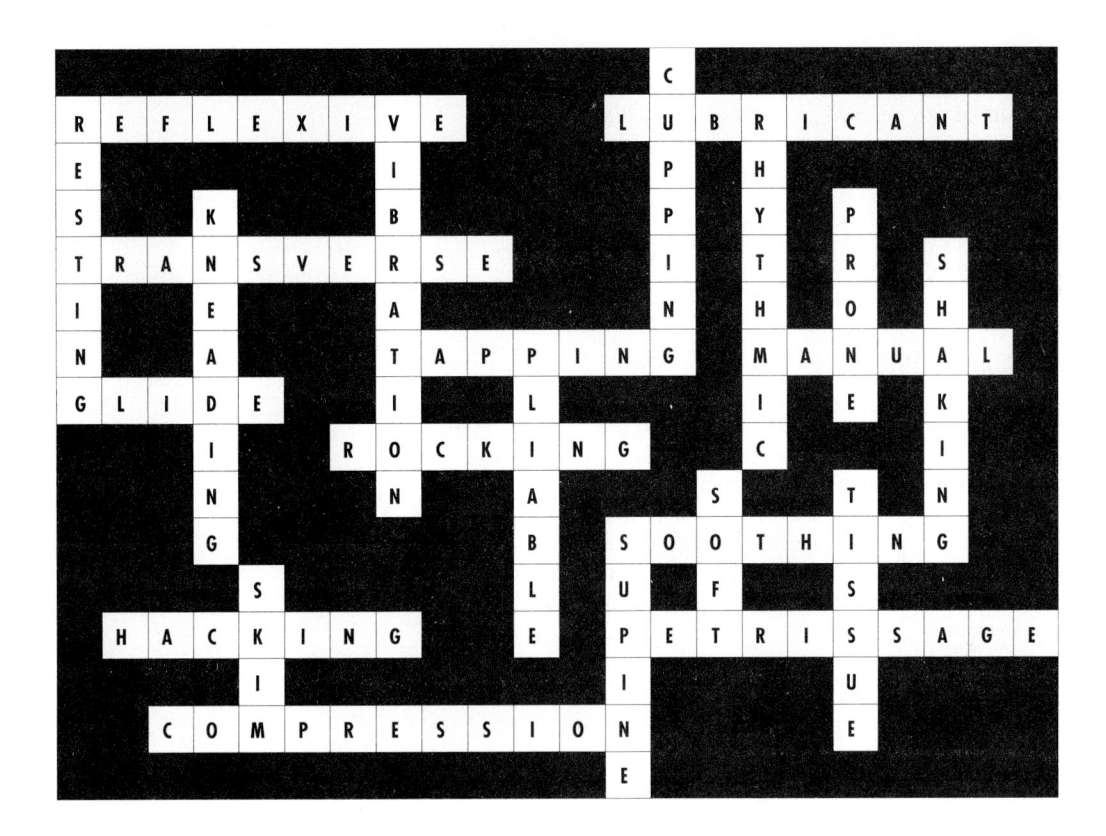

```
              C
R E F L E X I V E        L U B R I C A N T
E           I            P      H
S     K     B            P      Y     P
T R A N S V E R S E      I      T     R     S
I     E     A            N      H     O     H
N     A     T A P P I N G       M A N U A L
G L I D E   I            L      I     E     K
      I     R O C K I N G       C     T     I
      N     N     A             S     I     N
      G           B       S O O T H I N G
            S     L       U     F     S
          H A C K I N G   P E T R I S S A G E
            I     E       P           U
            C O M P R E S S I O N     E
            E
```

D. MATCHING

1. m
2. u
3. s
4. i
5. c
6. a
7. n
8. o
9. b
10. d
11. e
12. p
13. r
14. f
15. j
16. k
17. l
18. q
19. h
20. g
21. t

E. PROBLEM SOLVING EXERCISES

1. Muscle energy methods to produce lengthening would relax the muscle. Rocking of the body may relax the muscles.
2. Do compression and tapotement over a towel or sheet. The resting stroke can be used as can shaking, rocking and all massage techniques of joint movement, muscle energy, positional release, and lengthening and stretching approaches.
3. The entire body can be accessed in the other positions of supine, side-lying, and seated.

F. PROFESSIONAL APPLICATION

Reduce the amount of petrissage and tapotement and use it only when there is a specific purpose. Increase the muscle energy methods and lengthening. Increase the shaking and rocking methods. He should make sure that he is centered before giving the massage, and stretches his body afterwards. Check to see that the strokes are being applied with the correct body mechanics and he is making minimal use of his hands.

CHAPTER 11

Designing the Massage

A. KEY TERMS

Match the term to the best definition.

1. adaptation _____
2. application _____
3. assessment _____
4. body segment _____
5. fascial sheaths _____
6. gait _____
7. gesture _____
8. massage routine _____
9. mind-set _____
10. muscular tendinous junction _____
11. muscle testing procedures _____
12. objective assessment _____
13. open-ended question _____
14. palpation _____
15. plan/progress _____
16. phasic muscles _____
17. physical assessment _____
18. postural muscles _____
19. rapport _____
20. SOAP notes _____
21. subjective assessment _____
22. treatment plan _____

a. A general list of methods used, detail of any specific work, and the responses to the work. It is all recorded as part of the SOAP notes.

b. Where muscle fibers end and the connective tissue continues on to form tendon. Often a major site of injury.

c. Assessment process using muscle contraction. It may be used to determine strength, neurological interactions, or as an indicator of body function, similar to a biofeedback mechanism.

d. Information about what the next massage may include, things to remember to look for to re-evaluate the progress, a list of what seems to be working and not working, any self help that is shared, and other information that will influence future sessions.

e. Area of the body located between joints that provides for movement, especially during walking and balance.

f. Muscles that mainly move the body.

g. The development of a relationship based on mutual trust and harmony.

h. A method of charting and record keeping.

i. What the client provides as information during the interview and history-taking process and the client's goals and outcome for the session.

j. A shift in response to a sensory stimulation.

k. Total program for patient/client care developed by the physician or any member of the health care team.

l. The way people touch their bodies as they explain the problems, which could indicate a muscle, joint, or visceral problem.

m. Step-by-step protocol and sequence used to give a massage.

n. The collecting and interpretation of information provided by the client, the client's family and friends, the massage practitioner, and referring medical professionals.

o. Information and goals that the massage therapist gathers from the assessment process.

p. A way of phrasing a question so that the answer cannot be a simple one word response.

q. Assessment through touch.

r. Evaluation of body balance, efficient function, basic symmetry, range of motion, and ability to function.

s. Those muscles that support the body against gravity.

t. Flat sheets of connective tissue used for separation, stability, and muscular attachment points.

u. Preconceived idea that interferes with the ability to see alternatives.

v. Walking pattern.

B. FILL IN THE BLANKS

The first level of palpation does not include touching the body. It detects _____ and _____ areas. This is done best just off the skin using the _____ of the hand because the back of the hand is very sensitive to heat. Very sensitive cutaneous (skin) sensory receptors also detect changes in _____ and _____ of the air.

The second level of palpation is very light surface stroking of the _____. First, determine if the skin is dry or damp. The damp areas will feel a little sticky or the fingers will _____. This light stroking will also cause the _____ that senses light touch to respond. It is important to notice if any area gets more _____ than the other areas (pilomotor reflex). Although not palpation, this is a good time to _____ for color, especially blue or yellow coloration. The practitioner should also note and keep track of all _____ and surface skin growths, pay attention to the _____ and _____ of the hair, and observe the _____ and _____ of the nails.

The third level of palpation is the skin itself. This is done through small gentle, _____ of the skin in all directions and comparing the _____ of these areas. By applying light pressure to the skin surface, _____ or _____ can be felt. A method such as _____ or _____ is used to further assess the texture of the skin by lifting it from the underlying fascial sheath. The skin should move evenly and glide on the underlying tissues, and areas that are _____, _____, or too _____ should be noted. The fifth level of palpation is the superficial connective tissue. This layer of tissue is found by using _____ until the fibers of the underlying muscle are felt. The pressure should then be _____ so that if the hand is moved, the skin moves too, but the muscle cannot be felt. The tissue should feel _____ and _____ like gelatin. If there is surface edema, it will be in the _____.

Just above the muscle, and still in the superficial connective tissue, lie the more _____ blood vessels. The vessels are distinct and feel like _____. Pulses can be palpated, but if pressure is too _____, the feel of the pulse will be lost. Lymph nodes are usually located in _____ and feel like small, soft gelcaps. Muscle has a distinct _____ that can be felt. This texture feels somewhat like corded fabric or fine rope. When the muscle fibers end and the connective tissue continues, the _____ develops. There are often three or more _____ of muscle in an area. The layers usually run _____ to each other. Tendons have a higher concentration of elastin fibers and feel more _____ and less ribbed than muscle. Under many tendons is a fluid-filled ___ cushion that assists the movement of the bone under the tendon. Fascial sheathes separate muscle and expand the connective tissue area of bone for _____. Some run on the surface of the body, like the _____, the _____ and the _____. Others run _____ to the surface of the body and the bone, such as the _____ and the nuchal ligament. Still others run horizontal through the body. This occurs at _____, the diaphragm muscle (which is mostly connective tissue), and the pelvic floor. The larger _____ and _____ lie in the grooves created by the fascial separations. The ninth level is the ligaments. They are found around joints and are high in _____ and not very stretchy. Most assessment, at the basic massage level, is with _____. The sense should be a stable, supported, resilient, and unrestricted _____. With the joint movements, it is important to assess for _____. For the massage practitioner, it is important to be able to palate the _____ that indicate the tendinous attachment points for the muscles, and to be able to trace the bone shape. The _____ contains viscera or organs of the body.

The thirteenth level is the body rhythms, which are even pulsations. The three basic rhythms are the respiration, the blood, and the cranial-sacral rhythm.

Basic palpation of the breath is done by placing the hands over the _____ and allowing the body to go through three or more cycles as you evaluate the evenness and fullness of the breath. Basic palpation of the movement of the blood is done by placing the finger tips over _____ on both sides of the body and comparing for evenness. Basic palpation of the _____ is done by lightly placing the hands on either side of the head and sensing for the widening and narrowing of the skull. Also place a hand over the _____ and feel for the to-and-fro movement.

Phasic muscles will _____ jump into action when tested and they will tire out fast. Phasic muscles will _____ in response to postural muscle shortening. Phasic muscles become hypertonic.

The bottom line is this. The _____ knows his or her own body best. It is the job of the practitioner to _____ what the client says verbally, visually, through body language, in the tissues, and in the movement patterns. Only by listening, observing, and touching will the _____ begin to show, and then the solutions can be found for the individual. The therapist should not hesitate to ask for help and should _____ when the problem is bigger than the professional skills determined by the scope of practice for massage therapy.

C. PUZZLE

Complete the puzzle by filling in the spaces with the following words.

adaptation
assessment
body segment
charting
gait
gestures
muscle testing
objective
open ended
plan
rapport
routine
SOAP
subjective
treatment plan

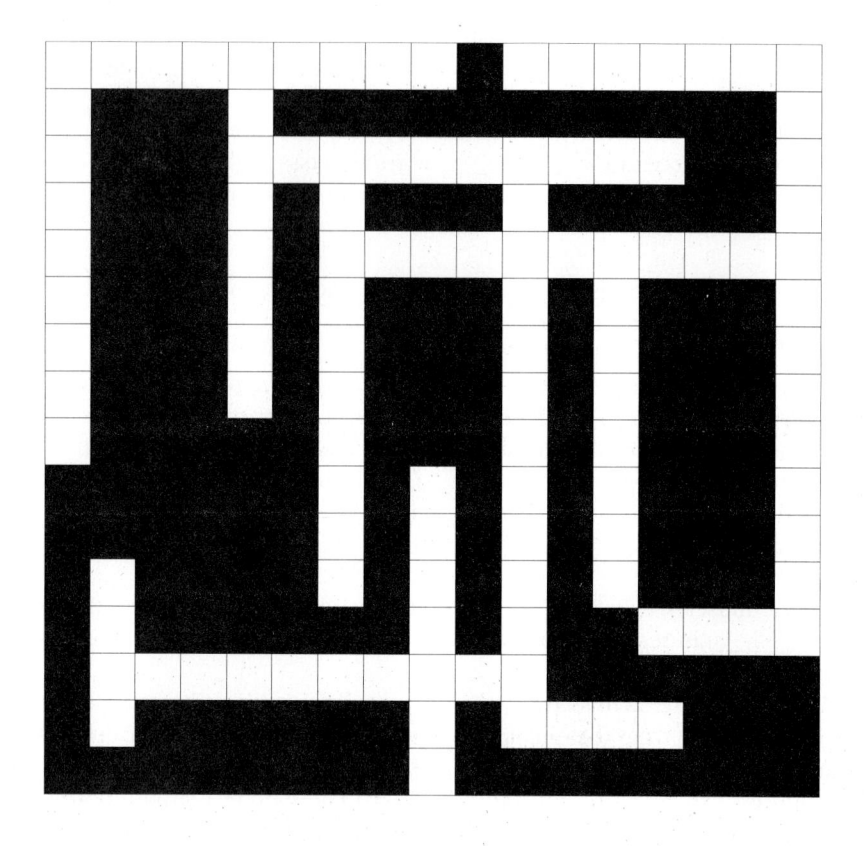

D. MATCHING

1. *The following statements apply to various massage manipulations. Choose the most correct answer or answers and match the strokes to the descriptions. Some responses may be used more than once.*

   a. The most common massage manipulation chosen is the effleurage/gliding stroke. This manipulation is effective for: _____

   b. Compression is effective for situations where: _____

   c. Rocking is very effective in the following situations: _____

   1. Applying lubricant
   2. A soothing approach for the massage
   3. Lubricant is not used
   4. People are hairy or ticklish
   5. The client prefers a more stimulating massage
   6. Excessive rubbing or pressing on the skin or underlying tissue is not desirable
   7. Clients desire a soothing massage with generalized body responses

2. *Match the muscle to its classification, depending on whether the muscle functions more by maintaining posture or moving us.*

Main Postural Muscles: A
Main Phasic Muscles: B

1. _____ Gastrocnemius			15. _____ Erector Spinae group
2. _____ Neck Flexors			16. _____ Pectorals
3. _____ Soleus			17. _____ Brachioradialis
4. _____ Adductors			18. _____ Latissimus Dorsi
5. _____ Deltoid			19. _____ Neck Extensors
6. _____ Medial Hamstrings			20. _____ Quadriceps
7. _____ Psoas			21. _____ Anterior Tibialis
8. _____ Biceps			22. _____ Trapezius
9. _____ Abdominal			23. _____ Hamstrings
10. _____ Rectus Femoris			24. _____ Gluteus Maximus
11. _____ Tensor Fascia Lata			25. _____ Scalene
12. _____ Piriformis			26. _____ Sternocleidomastoid
13. _____ Triceps			27. _____ Levator Scapula
14. _____ Quadratus Lumborum			

E. ADDITIONAL ACTIVITY

Doing the paperwork.

The following is a mock-up of a massage session, from initial interview to completion of the massage. Read the information given; then follow the instructions.

Sue Williams, a 37-year-old female client, is coming in for her first massage with you. She has received prior bodywork while a member of a health spa. She indicates that the massages were light and relaxing. At work, she is a middle management supervisor for a local manufacturing company. Her job requires time on the phone and many hours of meetings. The company is in the process of downsizing. She has been experiencing some tingling in her arms, and headaches, mainly at the back of her head. You notice that she squeezes her occipital area and pulls her hair in that location as she explains the headache. She has had some shortness of breath and lately has not been sleeping well. She did have a full physical check-up and nothing was found. Her doctor indicated that she was stressed and needed to find some ways to relax. Massage and exercise were given as options. She is in a long-term relationship and has two children, one 16 and one 9. She had a car accident 4 years ago with minor head trauma and whiplash. She broke her left ankle cheerleading in high school and tends to walk on the outside of that foot.

You notice that she also tends to roll her shoulders while breathing and sighs a lot. After a physical assessment, you find that she swings her left leg further than the right leg when walking and her right shoulder is high. She definitely is using shoulder muscles when she breathes. Her head is tilted towards her right shoulder. She seems to have a very mild kyphosis and is pulled forward in the chest area more so on the right so that there is a rotation at the thoracolumbar junction. There is limited movement in her right scapula and the right side of her ribcage. Palpation and muscle testing reveals that the tissue of the upper thorax is tight and restricted. Her lower leg muscles are tight, and her abdominals are weak.

You give a general massage using muscle energy methods to lengthen the shoulders, lower legs, and upper posterior neck. You explain to Sue that there is some connective tissue shortening in her upper chest and low back and posterior neck. Lengthening exercises are taught for the shoulders and lower leg. You suggest weekly massage for about six weeks and then a reevaluation.

Sue agrees and says that her headache is better but not entirely gone but she thinks she can breath better. Over all she feels more relaxed and wants to go home and take a nap.

After Sue leaves, you review her chart and wonder about the pattern between the broken ankle, whiplash, tight lower legs, shoulders, chest, and neck. You also wonder if wearing high heels may have something to do with the pattern as well as excessive sitting in meetings and talking on the phone.

Instructions:

Using this case study, complete the following Physical Assessment Form. It would help if you assumed the different postures as indicated in the information above and then assess yourself in a mirror. Complete the SOAP Notes Form that follows, using only the information given. Remember that much of this information is recorded on the client history form. Record only the information relevant for SOAP Notes.

PHYSICAL ASSESSMENT FORM

Complete Figure 11.1, the Physical Assessment Form.

PHYSICAL ASSESSMENT FORM			
Chin in line with nose, sternal notch, navel:	Yes	No	Explain
Shoulders:	Level	Left High/Right Low	Right Forward/Backward
	Right High/Left Low	Both Rolled Forward	Left Forward/Backward
Clavicles:	Level	Other	
Arms:	Hang Evenly	Left Rotated	How
	Right Rotated	How	Other
Elbows:	Even	Other	
Wrists:	Even	Other	
Fingertips:	Even	Other	
Ribs:	Even	Other	Springy
	Other		
Scapula: Move Freely	Yes	No	Explain
	Even	Other	
Abdomen:	Firm	Other	
Hard Areas:	Yes	No	Explain
Waist:	Level	Other	
Spine: Curves Normal	Yes	No	Explain
Gluteal Muscle Mass:	Even	Other	
Iliac Crest:	Even	Right High	Left High
Legs: Muscle Mass Even	Yes	No	Explain
Rotation:	Even	Other	
Trochanter:	Even	Other	
Knees:	Even	Other	
Patella: Movable	Yes	No	Even
	Other		
Ankles:	Even	Other	
Feet: Relaxed	Yes	No	Explain
Arches:	Even	Other	
Toes:	Explain		
Skin: Moves Freely	Yes	No	Explain
Pulls:	Yes	No	Explain
Puffy:	Yes	No	Explain

Fig. 11.1

SOAP NOTES STUDENT PRACTICE FORM

Complete Figure 11.2, the SOAP Notes Student Practice Form.

\	\	\	\	\	\
SOAP NOTES STUDENT PRACTICE FORM					
Date Name of Student	Practice Client's Name	Subjective Evaluation	Objective Evaluation	Application	Plan/ Progress
Techniques Used	Information Learned	Focus on Improvement for Next Session	What Worked Well	Client Comment	

Fig. 11.2

F. PROBLEM SOLVING EXERCISES

1. A client is obviously tense after a traffic tie up on the freeway. She is pacing and talking loud and fast. How would you begin the massage?

2. A client is complaining about a leg problem and showing you a spot on his knee. He keeps pointing to a particular area and drilling into the spot. What kinds of problems could be going on in that area?

3. A client has a damp area by her scapula that gets goose bumps when it is lightly touched. It also gets very red when massaged. What could be happening to cause these signs?

4. When comparing pulses in the foot you notice the right side is not as strong as the left side. The client says the right leg has been tingling. What should you do?

5. A factory worker has very tight trapezius and pectoralis muscles on the right side. His left hip has recently begun to ache and spasm. What might be going on?

G. PROFESSIONAL APPLICATION

You are being considered for a massage position with a chiropractor. The chiropractor wants to expand the wellness program that her office currently has and feels that massage would be a wonderful health service to offer. One of the things that is a major concern to all the current staff member is the ability of another person to work effectively as part of the team. How will assessment skills be a major influencing factor for this job?

H. RESEARCH FOR FURTHER STUDY

Research charting procedures and physical assessment forms for various other health professions and compare them to the SOAP notes procedure and physical assessment forms presented in this text.

ANSWERS

A. KEY TERMS

1. j
2. a
3. n
4. e
5. t
6. v
7. l
8. m
9. u
10. b
11. c
12. o
13. p
14. q
15. d
16. f
17. r
18. s
19. g
20. h
21. i
22. k

B. FILL IN THE BLANKS

hot
cold
back
air pressure
movement

skin
drag
root hair plexus
goose bumps
observe
moles
quality
texture
shape
condition

stretching
elasticity
roughness
smoothness
petrissage
skin rolling
stuck

restricted
loose
compression
lightened
resilient
springy
superficial fascia

superficial
soft tubes
intense
joint areas
fiber direction
tendon
layers
cross grain
pliable
bursa
muscular attachment
lumbar dorsal fascia
abdominal fascia
iliotibial band
perpendicular
linea alba

joints
nerves
blood vessels
collagen
active and passive joint movements
range-of-motion
end-feel
bony landmarks
abdomen

ribs
pulse points
cranial sacral rhythm
sacrum

quickly
weaken

client
understand
patterns
refer

Designing the Massage

C. PUZZLE

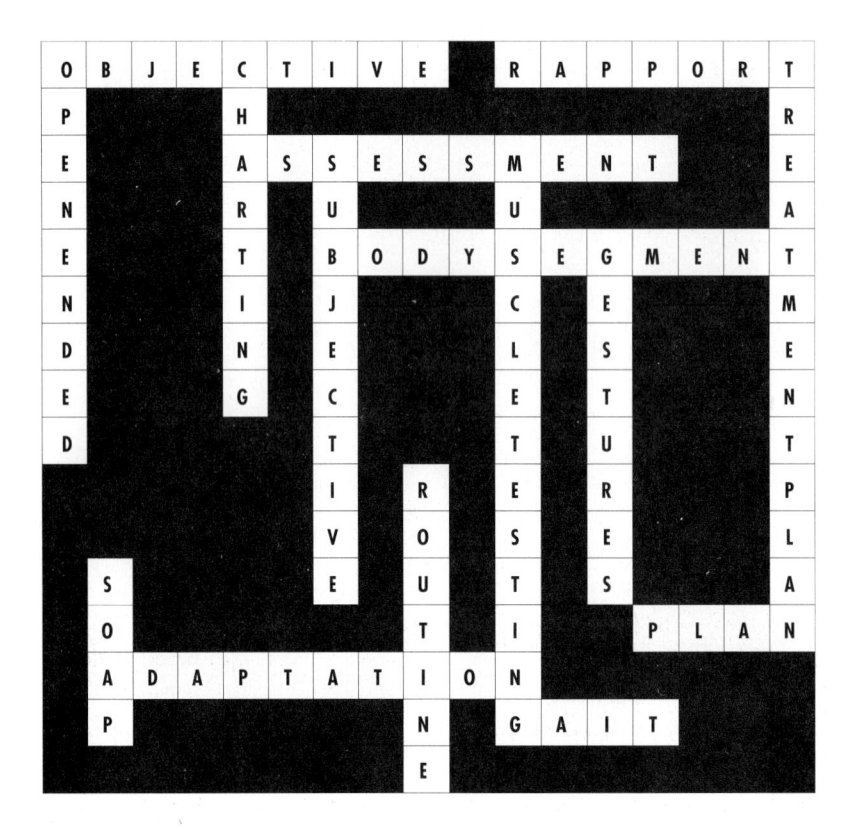

Across/Down answers filled in the crossword grid:

- OBJECTIVE
- RAPPORT
- PENNEENDED (vertical: P-E-N-N-E-N-D-E-D)
- HARTING (vertical: H-A-R-T-I-N-G)
- ASSESSMENT
- BODYSEGMENT
- SUBJECTIVE (vertical down from U-B-J-E-C-T-I-V-E)
- MUSCLETESTURES (vertical)
- TREATMENTPLAN (vertical)
- ROUTINE (vertical)
- SOAP
- ADAPTATION
- PLAN
- GAIT

D. MATCHING

1.

a. 1, 2
b. 3, 4, 5
c. 3, 4, 6, 7

2.

The following are B; the rest are A.
2, 5, 8, 13, 17, 20, 21, 23, 24

Chapter 11

E. ADDITIONAL ACTIVITY

PHYSICAL ASSESSMENT FORM			
Chin in line with nose, sternal notch, navel:	Yes	(No)	Explain Tilted to right
Shoulders:	Level	Left High/Right Low	(Right Forward/Backward)
	(Right High/Left Low)	Both Rolled Forward	Left Forward/Backward
Clavicles:	Level	(Other)	Right side higher
Arms:	Hang Evenly	Left Rotated	How
	(Right Rotated)	How	Other
Elbows:	Even	(Other)	Right side higher
Wrists:	Even	(Other)	Right side higher
Fingertips:	Even	Other	Right side higher
Ribs:	Even	(Other)	Springy
	Other	Right side does not move as free as left	
Scapula: Move Freely	Yes	(No)	Explain
	Even	Other	Right side not free moving
Abdomen:	Firm	(Other)	Muscles weak
Hard Areas:	Yes	(No)	Explain Mild kyphotic curve
Waist:	(Level)	Other	
Spine: Curves Normal	Yes	(No)	Explain
Gluteal Muscle Mass:	(Even)	Other	
Iliac Crest:	(Even)	Right High	Left High
Legs: Muscle Mass Even	(Yes)	No	Explain
Rotation:	(Even)	Other	
Trochanter:	(Even)	Other	
Knees:	(Even)	Other	
Patella: Movable	(Yes)	No	Even
	Other		
Ankles:	(Even)	Other	
Feet: Relaxed	(Yes)	No	Explain
Arches:	(Even)	Other	
Toes:	Explain		
Skin: Moves Freely	Yes	(No)	Explain Restriction at right upper thorax
Pulls:	Yes	No	Explain
Puffy:	Yes	No	Explain

E. ADDITIONAL ACTIVITY (cont.)

SOAP NOTES STUDENT PRACTICE FORM

Date Name of Student	Practice Client's Name	Subjective Evaluation	Objective Evaluation	Application	Plan/Progress
Fill in date and your name	Sue Williams	Tingling in arms Headaches-back of head squeezes occiput and pulls hair Shortness of breath Not sleeping well lately	Rolls shoulders while breathing Sighs a lot Left leg swings further while walking Rotation at thoracolumbar junction Palpation and muscle testing Shows: Tissues of upper thorax tight and restricted Lower leg muscles tight Abdominals weak	General massage muscle energy to lengthen shoulders, lower legs, and upper posterior neck	Suggest six weekly massage sessions, then re-evaluate Taught lengthening exercises for shoulders and lower legs
Techniques Used	Information Learned	Focus on Improvement for Next Session	What Worked Well	Client Comment	
Muscle energy		Increased stress reduction and relaxation		Headache better, but not gone Can breathe better Feels more relaxed	

F. PROBLEM SOLVING EXERCISES

1. In general, excessive sympathetic activation would be balanced by a relaxing massage, and excessive parasympathetic activation would be balanced by a stimulation massage. If the client is functioning from sympathetic nervous system control, and relaxation methods such as rocking and slow effleurage are initially used, the work will often be irritating. By beginning with a more stimulating approach, and using such strokes as rapid compression, PNF, stretching, and tapotement, the design of the massage fits where the client is physiologically. Once some of the nervous energy is discharged, the client is ready for the more relaxing methods.

2. A finger pointing to a specific area could suggest an acupressure or motor point hyperactivity, or a joint problem. What the pointing means depends on the area being pointed to. Because the client is drilling into a joint it may be wise to refer for joint dysfunction evaluation.

3. Damp areas on the skin show that the nervous system is activated in that area. This small amount of perspiration is part of a sympathetic activation called a facilitated segment. Surface stroking, with pressure enough to drag, will elicit a red response over the areas that are hyperactive. Deeper palpation will usually show a tender response. The small erector pili muscles attached to each hair are also under sympathetic autonomic nervous system control. Light fingertip stroking will produce goose-bumps over areas of hyperactivity.

4. Pulses should be compared by feeling for a strong, even, full pumping action on both sides of the body. If differences are perceived, a referral to the doctor is needed. Sometimes the differences in the pulses can be attributed to soft tissue restricting the artery, which will be determined by the physician.

5. A major problem is very likely hypertonic muscles. If shortened postural muscles are found, they need to be lengthened. If shortened and weak phasic muscles are located, they will first have to be lengthened and stretched. Eventually, strengthening techniques and exercises will be needed. If the hypertonic phasic muscle pattern is from repetitive use, the muscles will need to be fatigued with muscle energy/PNF techniques and then lengthened.

G. PROFESSIONAL APPLICATION

It will be important to both be able to understand the assessment procedures of chiropractic and be able to provide concise information to the chiropractor for evaluation in the development of a total treatment plan. The ability to keep clear, concise client SOAP notes will be valuable in comparing and coordinating the combined therapy.

CHAPTER 12

Special Populations

A. KEY TERMS

Match the term to the best definition.

1. barrier free _____
2. chronic illness _____
3. disability _____
4. dissociation _____
5. hospice _____
6. inter-competition massage _____
7. post-event massage _____
8. postpartum _____
9. pre-event massage _____
10. terminal _____
11. thermoregulator dysfunctions _____
12. trimester _____

a. Facilities and construction that provide access for those in wheelchairs and other mobility disabilities.
b. Illness of long duration.
c. Physical or mental condition resulting in some limitation or compromise in function.
d. Massage provided during an athletic event.
e. Massage provided after an athletic event.
f. After birth.
g. Three-month segments of a pregnancy
h. A coping mechanism that separates cognitive functions from physical feelings.
i. Massage provided before an athletic event.
j. Death is expected usually within a six month period.
k. An increase or decrease in internal body temperature.
l. Organization that provides specialized care for the terminally ill.

B. FILL IN THE BLANKS

It is the massage professional's responsibility to _____ as much as possible about the situation with which he or she is dealing. When people are abused, whatever the form of the abuse, they must learn to _____, as best they can, at the time of the abuse.

The technical term for this is state-dependent memory. This type of memory is _____ in the brain in a manner that includes the position, emotion, chemicals, nervous system activation, and all other combined physiology affecting the internal functions of a person at the time the experience happened. Some life experiences that may affect a person in a manner _____ to abuse are illness, medical procedures, hospitalization, accidents, and other trauma. The success of the individual's coping skills will depend on the type of _____ received during and soon after the event, as well as the dynamics surrounding the situation. The touch of the massage therapist may _____ the body of the abuse. If a client should respond during the massage by crying, shaking, becoming agitated, fearful, panicking, or through another emotional pattern, it is important for the massage professional to be still and let the person experience the emotion. If the client seems unsettled and needs additional coping help, he or she should be _____ to a qualified counselor.

Massage can be very beneficial for athletes if the massage professional understands the _____ required in the sport. If not, massage could _____ the optimum function of the athletic performance. If a massage professional plans to work with an athlete, it is important to know the person and become _____ of the training experience. The therapist should _____ about the sport, what is required of the athlete's body and mind, how to best use massage to enhance performance, and how to _____ the body in compensating patterns. If a massage professional is doing promotional work at sports massage events, working with many unfamiliar athletes, it is best to do _____ event massage. This way, the effects of any neurological disorganization caused by the massage are not _____. No connective tissue work, intense stretching, trigger points, or other _____ work should be done with an athlete at a sporting event.

This type of public, promotional environment is one area where following a sport massage _____ is important. The massage lasts about _____, and is quick-paced. It is important to watch for any _____ that could be a sign of sprains, strains, or compression fractures, and to refer the athlete to the medical tent for immediate evaluation. It is also important to watch for thermoregulatory disruption or hypo- and hyperthermia and _____ immediately.

Providing massage services for children is not much different than for _____. It is important that the practitioner _____ work with children and adolescents without parental or guardian supervision. The massage time can be used to _____ the parent or guardian some massage methods to use to help the child, and to teach the child some massage methods for use on the parent.

Dealing with chronic illness is difficult for the person who has it, for the doctor, and for the massage therapist. In many situations not much can be done except to make the day-to-day living with the illness more _____. The massage professional who wishes to work with the chronically ill needs to have _____ expectations. Massage can also _____ general stress levels by helping the individual to cope better with his or her condition. If the person is having a bad day, the massage should not be overdone. Those with a chronic illness often _____ activity levels, isolate themselves, and become less hardy. Massage, hydrotherapy, specially designed hardening programs, and exercise are ways of increasing a person's _____. It is important to work closely with the medical professionals involved to understand the effects of the various _____. Because massage does influence the physiology, there can be an _____ with the medication.

A resourceful goal for working with people with chronic illness is helping a client _____ the fact that each person is in charge of his or her own life, and the illness is not.

Chapter 12

People in their advanced years can greatly _____ from massage. Although the methods of massage are no _____, the elderly do present specific situations. Muscle tissue has _____ and been replaced by fat and connective tissue. Bones are not as flexible and are more prone to _____. Joints are worn and _____ is common. Skin is _____ and circulation is not as efficient. _____ may be prescribed to control blood pressure and other conditions. The interaction with a massage therapist provides both physical and emotional _____ for the elderly.

When working with any person, the massage professional needs to meet the person where he or she is at the _____. This is even more important when working with infants. If the parent or the massage practitioner expects the infant to _____ into the massage immediately, he or she may be disappointed. It is appropriate to _____ parents to massage their own babies.

People with a physical impairment can benefit from massage for all the _____ reasons as any other individual. In addition, dealing daily with a physical impairment can make _____ functions more stressful. The best source of information is the _____ with the impairment. The practitioner should use good judgment when deciding whether to _____ if assistance is needed, and then wait until the person accepts the offer before _____ assistance.

Informed _____ is a big concern with those who are influenced by drugs (both prescribed and not) internal chemicals, as well as developmental disabilities. Massage has a strong _____ effect on the autonomic nervous system. Those wishing to work with clients with mental impairments will need _____ training to be able to understand the physiology and psychology of the various disorders and challenges their clients face. This type of work should be _____ closely by a psychologist or psychiatrist.

Good, early prenatal care is very important for pregnant women. The massage professional must have _____ from the doctor or licensed midwife to work with a woman during this time. Deep work on the _____ is avoided, while surface stroking may be pleasurable. Alternate positioning for _____ or support for the abdomen is important.

In cases in which there is nothing more that can be done to prolong life, the focus of care is more on _____ measures. The experts in this situation of terminal illness are the dedicated hospice nurses and staff who treat death with _____. Being bedridden and Immobile is painful. Massage can distract the sensory perception and provide temporary comfort measures. It provides continued _____ contact, and can give care givers something useful, rewarding, and positive to do for their loved one who is dying. Massage can become an important stress reduction method and a means of support for _____ members and care givers.

C. PUZZLE

Complete the crossword puzzle by supplying answers to the following clues.

ACROSS:
1. Massage after a physical activity
6. Approaching the end
7. Physical or verbal attack or injury
8. Newborn
9. Those with a chronologic age above sixty
10. A specialized sense for recognition of sounds
12. A subjective emotional state
13. People from age three to eighteen
14. Providing for access for those with mobility disabilities

DOWN:
1. After the delivery of a newborn
2. A disorder affecting one or more of the body systems
3. A person who participates in sports
4. "Great expectations"
5. Before it happens
10. Organization providing specialized care for terminally ill
11. Long lasting, with slow progression or little change

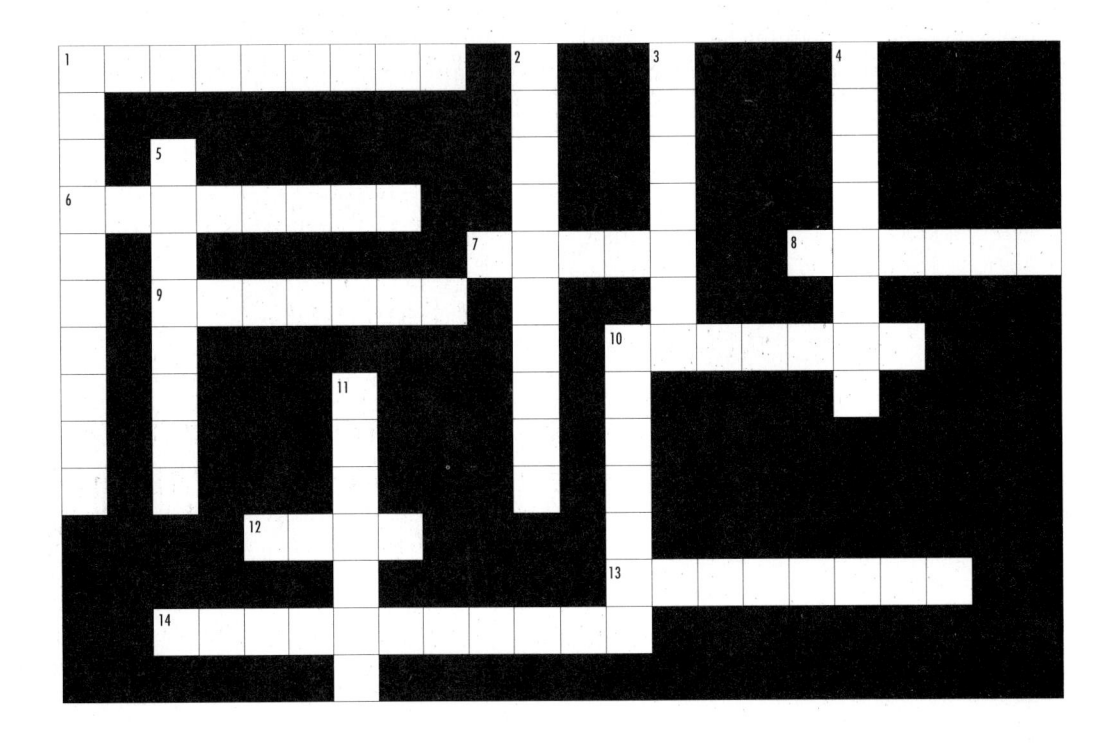

D. PROBLEM SOLVING EXERCISES

1. You are working at an organized sporting event as a volunteer to the local sports massage team. You notice that one of the other team members is doing deep invasive work on one of the clients. What should you do?

2. A client begins to shake and breath very deep during the massage. What do you do?

3. An elderly client wants you to stay after the massage and have a cup of coffee. What do you do?

4. A young father is having trouble holding his newborn baby. What can you do?

5. A client with a speech difficulty needs to provide informed consent. How could this be accomplished?

6. A client is near death. He does not want a full massage but does need to be touched. What can you do?

E. PROFESSIONAL APPLICATION

You are asked to give a presentation to a group of nurses at a local hospital. They are looking for ways to use massage in various outpatient situations. They need a general explanation of how massage would be beneficial in many different conditions. What major points would you make during the talk?

F. RESEARCH FOR FURTHER STUDY

A major approach for massage is generalized, nonspecific body supportive care. It does not seek to intervene but instead to provide support and nurture health. Brainstorm the various applications for massage in special needs situations and then find research to support some of the concepts.

ANSWERS

A. KEY TERMS

1. a
2. b
3. c
4. h
5. l
6. d
7. e
8. f
9. i
10. j
11. k
12. g

B. FILL IN THE BLANKS

learn	tolerable	same
survive	realistic	routine
	reduce	person
encoded	reduce	ask
similar	hardiness	providing
support	medication	
remind	interplay	consent
referred		normalizing
	rediscover	additional
biomechanics		supervised
impair	benefit	
part	different	permission
learn	decreased	abdomen
support	breaking	side-lying
post	osteoarthritis	
significant	thinner	comfort
invasive	Medications	dignity
	stimulation	human
routine		family
fifteen minutes	moment	
swelling	settle	
refer	teach	
adults		
never		
teach		

C. PUZZLE

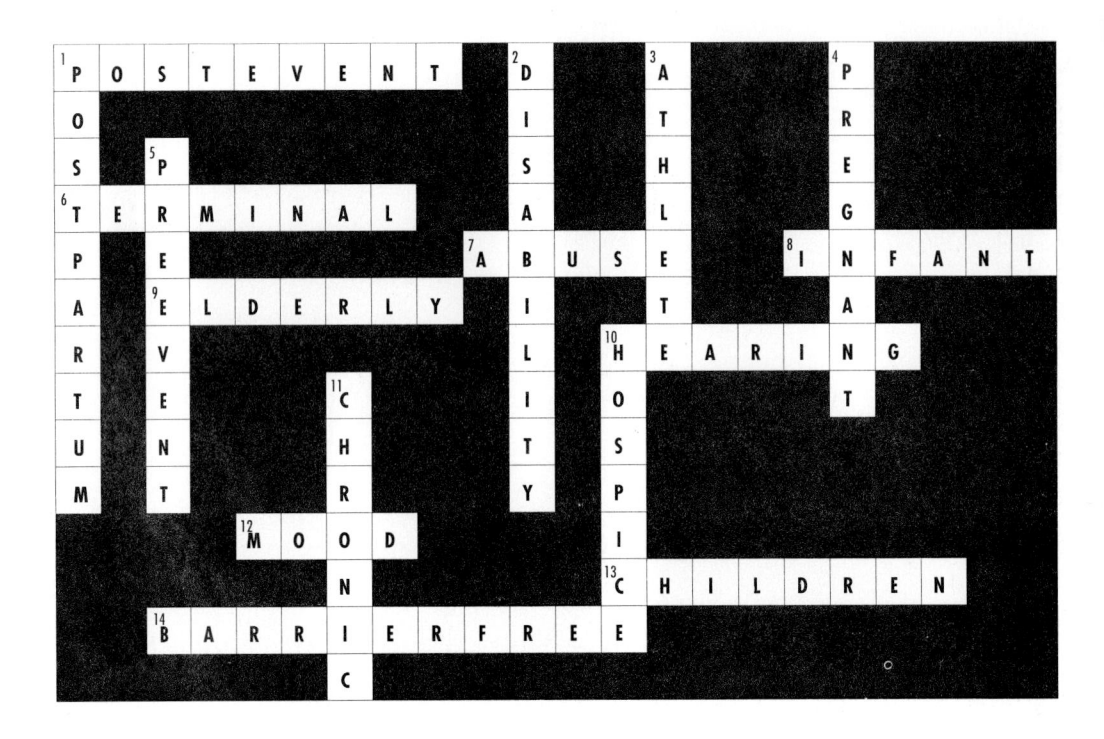

			¹P	O	S	T	E	V	E	N	T		²D			³A			⁴P			
			O										I			T			R			
			S		⁵P								S			H			E			
			⁶T	E	R	M	I	N	A	L			A			L			G			
			P		E					⁷A	B	U	S	E		E		⁸I	N	F	A	N	T
			A		⁹E	L	D	E	R	L	Y					T			A			
			R		V					I			¹⁰H	E	A	R	I	N	G			
			T		E			¹¹C		L			O			T						
			U		N			H		I			S									
			M		T			R		T			P									
							¹²M	O	O	D			I									
								N					¹³C	H	I	L	D	R	E	N		
			¹⁴B	A	R	R	I	E	R	F	R	E	E									
								C														

D. PROBLEM SOLVING EXERCISES

1. This is inappropriate behavior and could cause injury to the client. Either speak with the sports massage team leader or quietly ask to speak with the person and remind him that invasive work is inappropriate and could cause harm.

2. Gently ask the client if she is comfortable and if she would like to continue with the massage. If she would like to end the session, do so gently and with a sense of closure. If she chooses to continue, stay general with the approach and be quietly supportive.

3. This is a judgment call. Acknowledge that the social aspect of the massage is very important and if you choose to stay for a bit more conversation, realize that you are establishing a pattern that may need to be continued.

4. Teach him massage to provide a way to organize the touch and meet the needs of the infant.

5. The client can write the message or use other technology such as a voice synthesizer to communicate.

6. Gentle stroking of the hands and feet, and listening.

E. PROFESSIONAL APPLICATION

Massage is a good support for comfort care.
Massage is good for symptomatic relief of pain.
Massage evens the mood.
Massage reduces general stress levels.

CHAPTER 13

Basic Therapeutic Approaches

A. KEY TERMS

Match the term to the best definition.

1. acupressure _____
2. cryotherapy _____
3. hydrotherapy _____
4. myofascial release _____
5. reflexology _____
6. shiatsu _____
7. systemic massage _____
8. trigger point _____
9. yang _____
10. yin _____

a. The portion of the whole realm of function of the body, mind, and spirit of eastern thought that corresponds with parasympathetic autonomic nervous system functions.

b. The portion of the whole realm of function of the body, mind, and spirit of eastern thought that corresponds with sympathetic autonomic nervous system functions.

c. An area of local nerve facilitation resulting in hypertonicity of a muscle bundle and referred pain patterns.

d. Therapeutic use of various types and temperatures of water applications.

e. Methods used to tone or sedate acupuncture points without the use of needles.

f. The therapeutic use of ice.

g. Massage primarily structured to affect one body system. This approach is usually used for lymphatic and circulation enhancement massage.

h. A system of bodywork that affects the connective tissue of the body through various methods which elongate and alter the plastic component and ground matrix of the connective tissue.

i. A massage system directed primarily to the feet and hands.

j. An acupressure and meridian focused bodywork system.

B. FILL IN THE BLANKS

Hydrotherapy is a separate and distinct form of therapy that combines well with massage. Water's three forms (liquid, steam, and _____), allow for use in a variety of temperatures. The effects of water are primarily _____ and focused to the autonomic nervous system. In general, _____ stimulates sympathetic responses and _____ activates parasympathetic responses.

One of the most documented benefits of massage is stimulation of the lymphatics and _____. When the massage is focused to stimulate specifically the lymphatic or circulatory system, a special type of massage is performed. Because an entire body system is being stimulated, the approach is called _____ massage. The _____ system is a specialized component of the circulatory system, responsible for waste disposal and immune response. It moves from the interstitial space into the lymph capillaries though a pressure mechanism exerted by respiration, the _____ of muscles, and the pull of the skin and fascia during movement. This action is especially prominent at the plexuses in the _____ and feet. The pressure provided by massage _____ the compressive forces of movement and respiration.

_____ massage is focused specifically to stimulate the efficient flow of blood through the body. This type of massage tends to normalize blood pressure, tone the cardiovascular system, and undo the ill effects of occasional stress. Both circulatory and lymphatic massage are very beneficial for the client who is _____ to walk or exercise aerobically, whatever the reason. Massage to encourage blood flow to the tissues (arterial circulation) and then back to the heart (venous circulation) is _____. Because of the valve system of the veins and lymph vessels, any deep stroking over these vessels, from proximal to distal (from the heart out) is _____. There is small chance of breaking down the _____. However, _____, which does not slide like effleurage or stripping, is appropriate for stimulating arterial circulation. The short effleurage stroke is about three inches long and moves the blood from valve to valve. Long effleurage strokes carry the blood though the entire _____.

In the bodywork community, _____ is taken to mean the stimulation of areas beneath the skin to improve the function of the whole body or of specific body areas that are away from the site of the stimulation. The medical definition of reflexology is "the study of _____." There are many nerve endings on the feet and hands that _____ with acupressure points, which, when stimulated, trigger the release of _____ and other endogenous chemicals. In addition, major plexuses for the _____ system are located in the hands and feet. Compressive forces in this area would _____ lymphatic movement.

An excellent way to massage the foot is to systematically apply pressure and movement to the _____ foot and ankle complex. The pressure will stimulate the circulation, nerves, and _____. Moving all of the joints stimulates large-diameter nerve fibers and joint kinesthetic receptors, initiating hyperstimulation _____. The result is a shift in proprioceptive and postural _____.

The basic connective tissue approach consists of _____ softening the tissue through pressure, pulling, movement, and stretch on the tissues, which allows them to rehydrate and remold. The intent of connective tissue massage is to either to soften the ground matrix, or to introduce small amounts of _____, which triggers connective tissue restructuring. It is often futile to try to figure out connective tissue patterns.

_____ therapy is the umbrella encompassing a variety of treatment approaches, one of which is trigger point therapy. Trigger point therapy is one of many techniques found to be useful in the treatment of _____ problems. A trigger point is an area of local _____ facilitation of a muscle and is aggravated by stress of any sort affecting the body or the mind of the individual.

Acupuncture can be defined as the stimulation of certain points with needles inserted along the meridians (channels) and "AhShi" (trigger) points outside the meridians. **Acupressure** is a modified version of acupuncture that substitutes pressure for needle insertion. The oriental perspective considers at body functions in terms of balance between **opposing** forces. The pairing of **meridians** is called yin/yang. Yin meridians are associated with the **parasympathetic** autonomic nervous system responses and functions of the solid organs essential to life. Yang meridians are associated with the **sympathetic** autonomic nervous system responses and hollow organs whose functions are supportive to life, but not essential. Acupressure points usually lie in a **natural** division between muscles and near origins and insertions. Unlike a trigger point, which may only be found on one side of the body, acupressure points are **bilateral** (located on both sides of the body). To stimulate a hypoactive or "not enough" acupressure point, use a short vibrating or **tapping** action. To **sedate** a hyperactive or "too much" point for pain reduction, elicit the pain response within the point itself and use a sustained holding pressure until the painful over-energy dissipates and the body's own pain killers are released into the blood stream.

C. PUZZLE

This is a game that uses a special code. Key words from this chapter have been "translated" into a different alphabet. Once you find what one letter stands for, use that code for this entire puzzle.

The first word is given to you to help you get started.

1. pomravyymav — acupressure

So, in this puzzle, p stands for a, o stands for c, m stands for u, r stands for p, and so on.

2. oahlgdvaprh — cryotherapy
3. dhtalgdvaprh — hydrotherapy
4. jhlcpyoepw avwvpyv — myofascial release
5. avcwvklwluh — reflexology
6. yhygvjeo jpyypuv — systemic massage
7. ydepgy — shiatsu
8. gaeuuva rlefg — trigger point
9. hpfu — yang
10. hef — yin

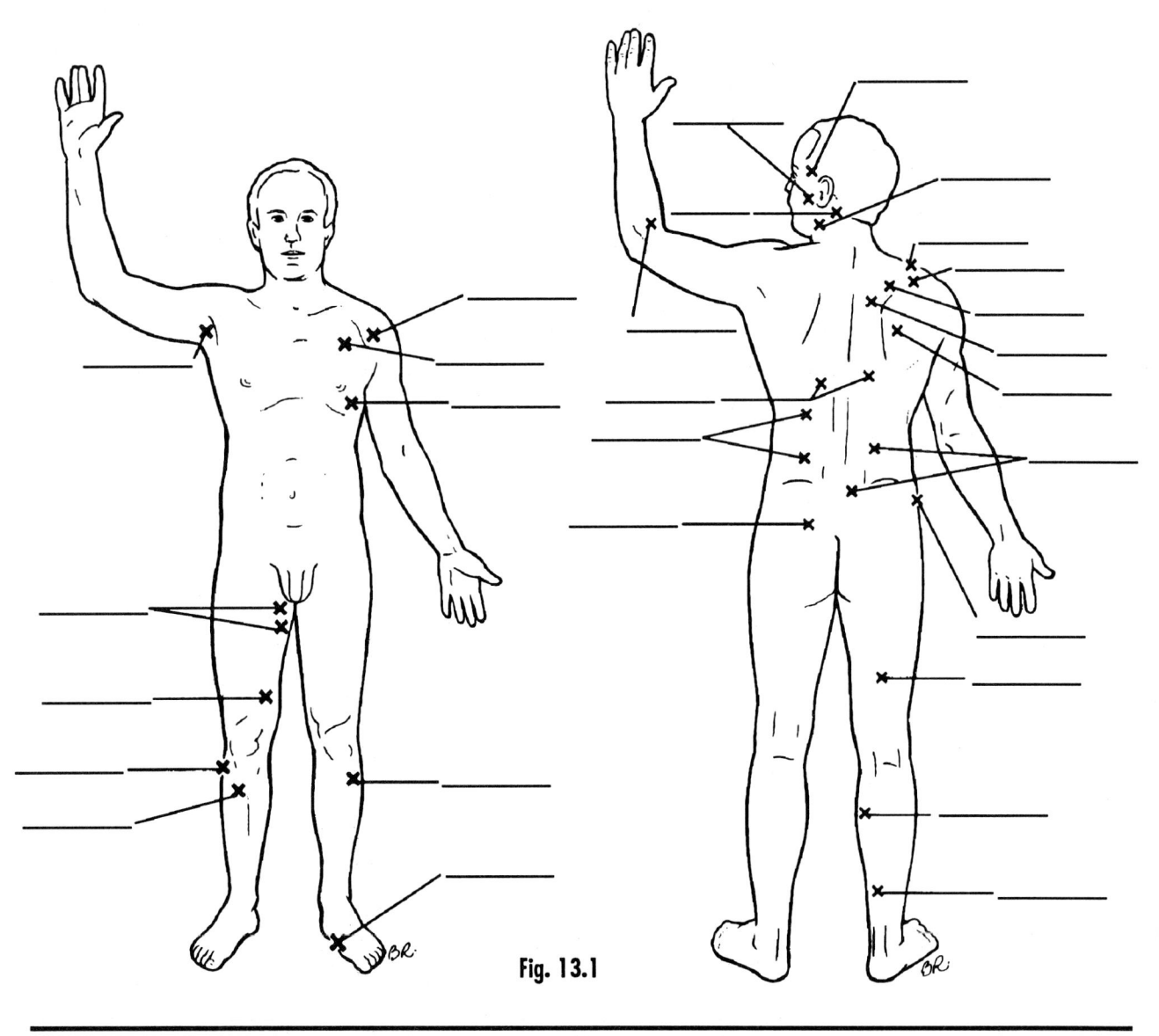

D. LABELING

Label the correct muscle names to show the locations of common trigger points in Figure. 13.1.

abductor hallucis	levator scapula	sternocleidomastoid
adductor longus	long extensors	subscapularis
anterior serratus	longissimus	supinators
biceps femoris	masseter	supraspinatus
deltoid	multifidus	temporalis
gastrocnemius	pectoralis	tibialis anterior
gluteus medius	peroneus longus	trapezius
gluteus minimus	soleus	upper trapezius
iliocostalis	splenius capitis	vastus medialis
infraspinatus		

Fig. 13.1

Chapter 13

E. MATCHING

1. When using hydrotherapy, the effects of the various forms and temperatures must be known so that the desired results can be achieved. Read the results on the left side, then place an 'X' in the correct columns to match with proper form and temperature. Some of the effects will show up in more than one answer.

	Effects of Heat	Effects of Cold	Effects of Ice
1. Increased circulation			
2. Decreased circulation			
3. Increased metabolism			
4. Decreased metabolism			
5. Increased stimulation			
6. Increased inflammation			
7. Decreased inflammation			
8. Decreased pain			
9. Decreased muscle spasm			
10. Decreased tissue stiffness			
11. Increased tissue stiffness			
12. Increased muscle tone			

2. Various reflexes are associated with the feet. Match the reflex with the description.

   1. Achilles tendon reflex
   2. extensor thrust
   3. flexor withdrawal
   4. Mendel-Bekhterev
   5. postural reflex
   6. Rossolimos reflex
   7. proprioceptive

a. Plantar flexion/extension of the foot resulting from contraction of calf muscles following a sharp blow to the Achilles tendon. Similar to the knee jerk reflex.

b. Flexion of the lower extremity when the foot receives a painful stimulus.

c. Plantar flexion of the toes in response to percussion of the dorsum of the foot.

d. A quick and brief extension of a limb upon application of pressure to the plantar surface.

e. Reflex initiated by movement of the body to maintain the position of the moved part. Any reflex initiated by stimulation of a proprioceptor.

f. Any reflex that is concerned with maintenance of posture.

g. Plantar flexion of second to fifth toes in response to percussion of plantar surface of the toes.

F. ADDITIONAL ACTIVITY

Determine which of these rules of hydrotherapy are false. Draw a line through each false statement.

1. Always take a thorough case history to check for possible contraindications. Contraindications include various circulatory and kidney problems, as well as skin conditions.

2. Always adapt the method to the individual and not the other way around. The procedures given for time length, temperatures used, etc., are to be used as guidelines and not absolutes.

3. Have the client go to the bathroom before treatment begins.

4. Leave the client totally alone for the duration of the treatment

5. Explain the complete treatment to the client only after the session is done.

6. Make sure the room is draft-free, clean, and quiet. All equipment should be sanitary and in good working condition. Each client should have clean towels and sheets.

7. Keep the client from becoming chilled during or after the treatment.

8. When using cold temperatures, the water should be as cold as possible, within the tolerance of the client. A 10° difference is the minimum needed to create stimulation and change in the circulation.

9. Warm temperatures should be as hot as the client can stand without causing discomfort.

10. More is NOT better. It is not always more effective to use greater extremes in temperature or greater lengths of time. The aim is to achieve a positive change, and too much can overtax, damage, or set back the condition.

11 Do not ask any question during the treatment.

12. Check the client's pulse before, during, and after treatments as required, especially with prolonged hot treatments. The pulse should stay fairly even.

13. Watch for discomfort and/or negative reactions to the treatment.

14. Do not stop the treatment if the client complains.

15. Generally, short cold treatments are followed by active exercise. Both prolonged cold and hot treatments are followed by bed rest, and then exercise.

16. Apply cold compresses to the head with both hot treatments and prolonged cold treatments.

17. It is okay to give a cold treatment to a cold body.

G. PROBLEM SOLVING EXERCISES

1. How can you tell the difference between a trigger point and an acupressure point?

   _____
   _____
   _____
   _____

2. A client wants a general relaxation massage but does have some mild circulation sluggishness. What style of massage would you use to best serve the client?

   _____
   _____
   _____
   _____

H. PROFESSIONAL APPLICATION

You are a massage therapist who has been in practice for about three years. An increasing number of your clientele seems to have connective tissue problems. What types of continuing education would help you to work most efficiently with these clients?

_____
_____
_____
_____

I. RESEARCH FOR FURTHER STUDY

How is hydrotherapy used in the physical therapy setting?

_____
_____
_____
_____

ANSWERS

A. KEY TERMS

1. e
2. f
3. d
4. h
5. i
6. j
7. g
8. c
9. b
10. a

B. FILL IN THE BLANKS

ice
reflexive
cold
warmth

circulation
systemic
lymph
compression
hands
mimics

Circulatory
unable
different
contraindicated
valves
compression
vein

reflexology
reflexes
correlate
endorphins
lymph
stimulate

entire
reflexes
analgesia
reflexes

mechanically
inflammation

Neuromuscular
myofascial
nerve

Acupuncture
Acupressure
opposing
meridians
parasympathetic
sympathetic
fascial
bilateral
tapping
sedate

C. PUZZLE

a. acupressure
b. cryotherapy
c. hydrotherapy
d. myofascial release
e. reflexology
f. systemic massage
g. shiatsu
h. trigger point
i. yang
j. yin

D. LABELING

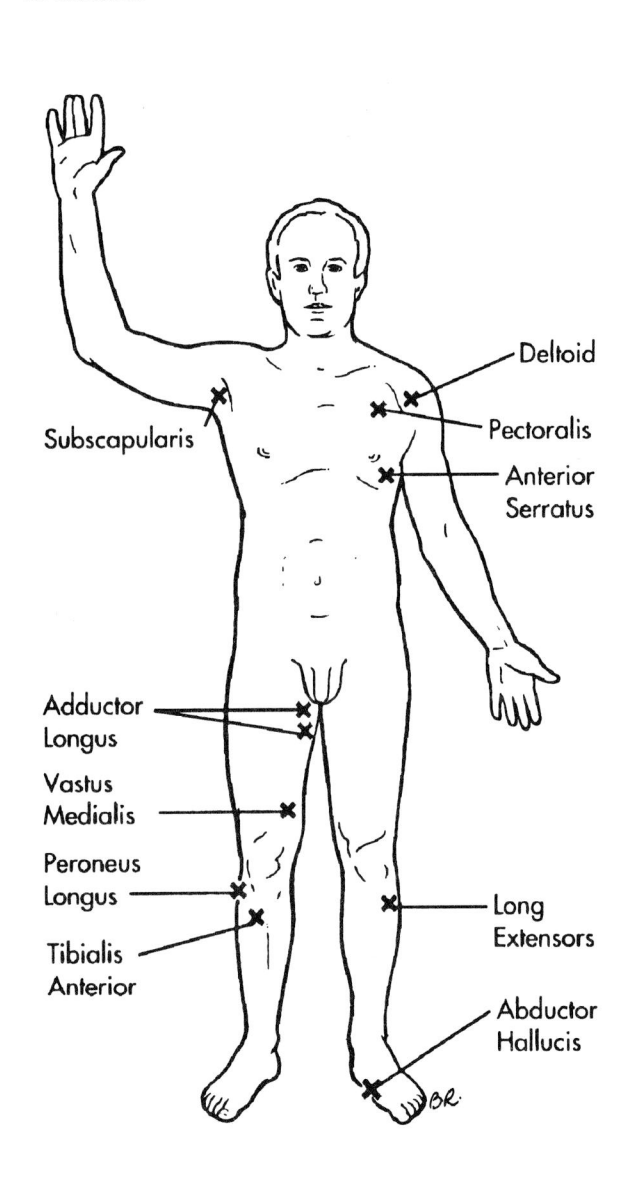

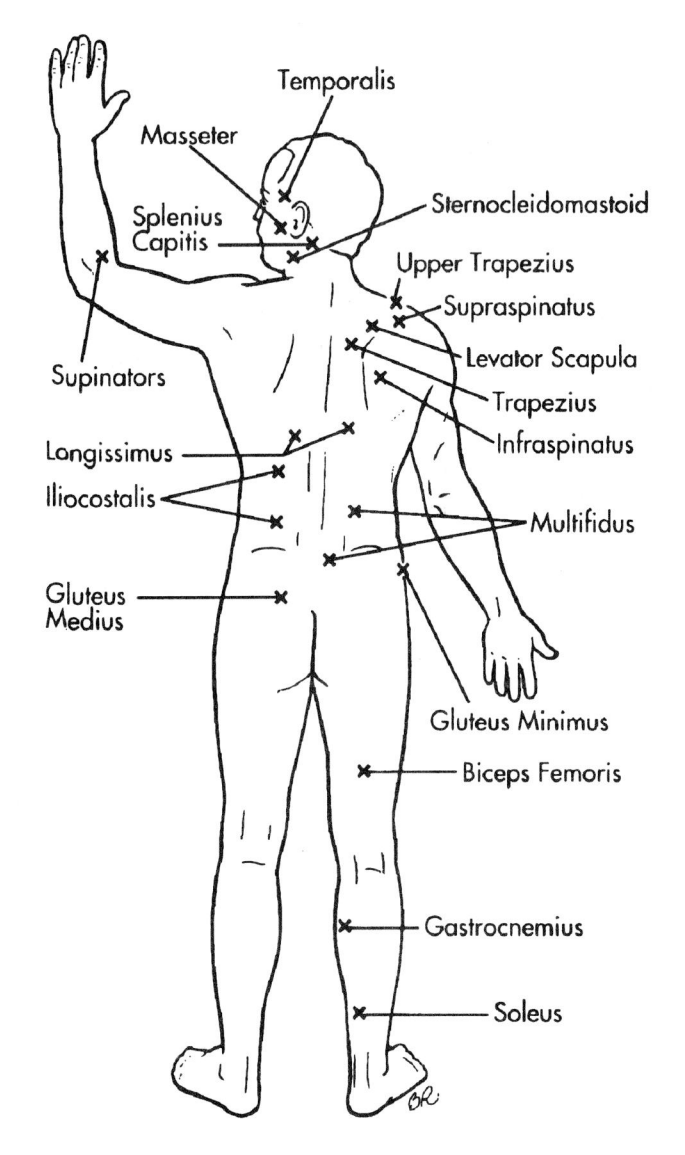

E. MATCHING

1.
Heat 1, 3, 6, 8, 9, 10
Cold 1, 5, 7, 8, 11, 12
Ice 2, 4, 7, 8, 9, 11

2.
1. a
2. d
3. b
4. c
5. f
6. g
7. e

F. ADDITIONAL ACTIVITY

False statements - 4, 5, 11, 14, 17

G. PROBLEM SOLVING EXERCISE

1. Acupressure points are bilateral. You should be able to find the same spot on the other side of the body. Trigger points usually are only on one side of the body.
2. Focus compression methods initially over the main arteries and then switch to effleurage strokes and joint movement for the major portion of the remainder of the massage.

H. PROFESSIONAL APPLICATION EXERCISE

Classes in trigger point therapy, deep transverse friction, myofascial release, and cranial-sacral therapy.

CHAPTER 14

Wellness Education

A. KEY TERMS

Match the term to the best definition.

1. hardiness _____
2. lifestyle _____
3. resourceful _____
4. stress _____
5. wellness _____

   a. Collection of behaviors.
   b. Clever and imaginative way of dealing with a situation that results in a desirable outcome.
   c. The efficient balance of body, mind, and spirit all working in a harmonious way providing for quality life.
   d. Resourceful coping style that includes commitment, internal sense of control, and perceiving change as a challenge.
   e. Any perception that causes the body to respond and adapt.

B. FILL IN THE BLANKS

We are considered _____ when body, mind, and spirit are in ideal balance. It does not seem to be just the type of stress, but rather the _____ of stress that accumulates until the breakdown begins. It is our _____ reaction to stress that may be the difference between positive action and destructive breakdown, especially if many of these stresses seem _____ our control. The three major elements of stress are the stressor itself, the _____ measures, and the mechanisms for surrender. Stressors are any internal perception or external stimuli that demand a _____ of the body. The _____ measures are how our bodies defend against the stressor. It is important and resourceful to know when to _____.

An _____ diet is low in fats and sugars and moderately low in protein and dairy with the bulk of the calories coming from complex carbohydrates. Drinking enough pure _____ is very important to a wellness program.

Slow, deep breathing takes _____. The shoulders do not move during _____ relaxed breathing. The accessory muscles of respiration located in the neck area should only be activated when _____ oxygen is required for fight or flight response. This is the pattern for _____ breathing. If the person does not balance the oxygen/carbon dioxide levels through increased activity levels, _____ may occur. Patterns of hyperventilation can perpetuate _____ states.

Exercise replaces movements lost by _____. General recommendations include _____ minutes daily of moderate aerobic activity, which _____ heart and breathing rates. Muscles and bones need to work against a load or weight to remain healthy, so _____ or weight training of some sort is also needed. Slow _____ can replace the bending and reaching that our bodies are designed for. Frequent five-minute stretches and breathing breaks should be built into everyone's day, especially for those who maintain _____ positions.

Relaxation methods initiate a _____ response. The most successful relaxation methods _____ movement, stretching, and tensing and then releasing muscles (progressive relaxation). The heart and breathing rate are _____ while focusing on a quiet or neutral topic, event, or picture. Almost any type of pleasurable, simple, repetitive activity that requires focused attention will induce the _____ response.

Feelings are the body's interpretation of _____. They occur as a response to the effect of hormones, neurotransmitters, and other endogenous _____. People use chemical substances like food, nicotine, alcohol, and drugs, to create _____. _____ such as creating crises, eating disorders, accident proneness, hypervigilance, panic, illness, depression, and codependent relationships can be used to change mood and feelings. Often, if the person's _____ can be changed, his or her feelings can also be changed. The easiest way to change the physiology is to _____, as in exercising or breathing. A massage will also change the _____.

_____ are feelings driven by thoughts and actions. As humans, we _____ to be helpless, addictive, and have low self esteem. The important point to remember is that if we learned the maladaptive behavior in the first place, we can also learn a more _____ behavior to use instead.

_____ is what we do in response to feelings, to trigger feelings, and occasionally to avoid feelings. Resourceful behavior results in a good feeling and feeling _____ about what happened. Unresourceful behavior still results in a good feeling (or we wouldn't do it), but often we feel _____ about what happened, and/or others feel bad. It takes hard work and lots of _____ to change an addictive behavior. Instead of basing our value on an external standard, people who are well will develop _____ standards of self worth.

Resourceful _____ consists of commitment, control, and challenge. Poor stress-coping skills and unresourceful emotions are immune _____ and predispose us to infection and poor health. It is the individual's _____ to the stress that determines the effect of immunity, not the stress itself. Wellness includes learning more efficient ways to _____ with life.

Faith is the ability to_____, trust and know certain things that science cannot prove. Hope is the belief, assurance, conviction, and confidence that our future will somehow be _____. Without love there is no wholeness and without wholeness there is no _____. Success is the _____ utilization of the abilities you have. All great achievements require time, _____, and purpose. Massage brings an _____ of body, mind, and spirit. Most importantly, massage touches _____, and in turn, we are touched by them.

C. PUZZLE

Find the following words in the word search.

- behavior
- body
- breathing
- commencement
- coping
- emotions
- exercise
- faith
- feelings
- hardiness
- hope
- know thyself
- lifestyle
- love
- mind
- nutrition
- relaxation
- resourceful
- self-concept
- spirit
- stress
- stretching
- wellness

```
W E L L N E S S H G F D C B A E
C O M M E N C E M E N T S F G M
L I F E S S T L Y F E H T J K O
B M N O T G Y D O B A I R P Q T
O R U R N C H J N V R I E K N I
W E E I P Q R O S I E T T U O O
N S P A V W X Y P Z M A C H I N
S O H O T A I S L E Y P H R T S
C U R Y C H R I O M A S I B A H
A R U N N O I T I R T U N S X A
T C A D F G J N F K N Q G I A R
F E E L I N G S G B L U E S L D
J F R S T L E E S I C R E X E I
K U B E H A V I O R S T Y G R N
F L E S Y H T W O N K K N N O E
R A M O U T P E C N O C F L E S
L I F E S T Y L E R I C H A N S
```

D. ADDITIONAL ACTIVITY

List 15 common stress responses:

1. _____
2. _____
3. _____
4. _____
5. _____
6. _____
7. _____
8. _____
9. _____
10. _____
11. _____
12. _____
13. _____
14. _____
15. _____

E. PERSONAL APPLICATION

1. Write your history. Include your physical and mental health story, family history, and any details that jump out—both pleasant and unpleasant. Write down dates and as many details as possible. Talk with family and friends. Look through photo albums, watching for sign of stress in the pictures.

_____
_____
_____
_____
_____
_____
_____
_____
_____
_____
_____
_____
_____
_____

2. Clarify one miscommunication with a classmate, learning partner, friend, or family member that occurred during your study of massage. Relate this to stress/wellness.

3. From all the sources you have ever encountered regarding wellness information, list your experts and resource books. Make sure you have three from each category of nutrition, breathing, exercise, stretching, relaxation methods, feelings, emotions, behavior, self-concept, coping mechanisms, faith, hope, and love.

4. List three fundamental wellness truths you learned about yourself during the study of this chapter.

5. Using the model for a business plan, develop a generalized personal wellness plan. Include both a mission statement and motivation statement about wellness.

   _____
   _____
   _____
   _____
   _____
   _____
   _____
   _____

6. Decide what part of wellness is hard work for you; list this difficulty.

   _____
   _____
   _____
   _____

7. Pick one small lifestyle change and take two days to prepare to make the change. List the change as well as the necessary preparations.

   For example: Life style change: walk for 30 minutes three times a week. Preparations: buy new walking shoes, figure out walking route, schedule time of day to walk.

   _____
   _____
   _____
   _____

8. Design a 15 minute self-help exercise and stretching program, focusing on your specific needs. List your routine.

   _____
   _____
   _____
   _____

9. List three areas of consideration or special attention you will need help with as you set up your personal wellness program.

   _____
   _____
   _____
   _____

10. Share with one person how your spiritual self, whatever that is to you, has emerged while studying massage. Also share why massage is a part of this awareness.

    _____
    _____
    _____
    _____

ANSWERS

A. KEY TERMS

1. d
2. a
3. b
4. e
5. c

B. FILL IN THE BLANKS

well	parasympathetic	coping
amount	combine	suppressing
emotional	synchronized	response
beyond	relaxation	cope
defensive	emotions	
change	chemicals	believe
defensive	feelings	OK
quit	Behaviors	wellness
	physiology	maximum
ideal	move	perseverance
water	physiology	awareness
		people
time	Emotions	
normal	learn	
increased	resourceful	
sympathetic		
hyperventilation	Behavior	
anxiety	good	
	bad	
inactivity	support	
30	internal	
increases		
resistance		
stretching		
static		

C. PUZZLE

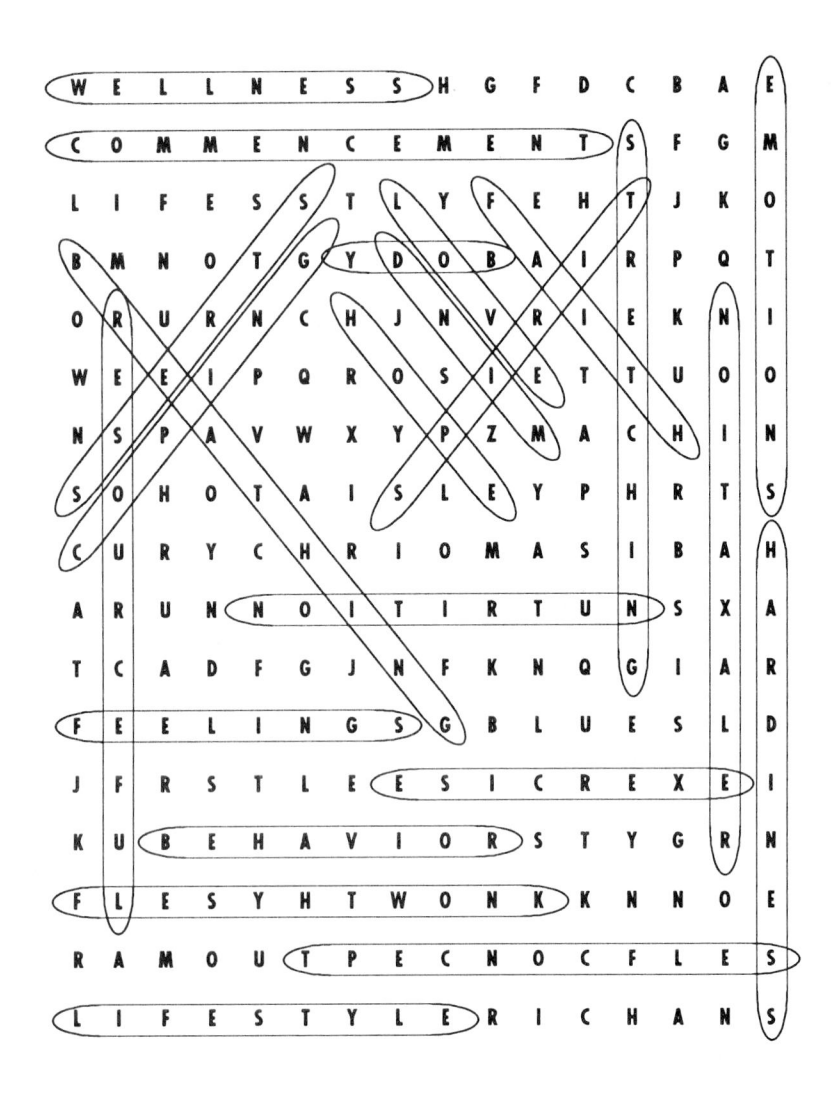

```
W E L L N E S S H G F D C B A E
C O M M E N C E M E N T S F G M
L I F E S S T L Y F E H T J K O
B M N O T G Y D O B A I R P Q T
O R U R N C H J N V R I E K N I
W E I P Q R O S I E T T U O O
N S P A V W X Y P Z M A C H I N
S O H O T A I S L E Y P H R T S
C U R Y C H R I O M A S I B A H
A R U N N O I T I R T U N S X A
T C A D F G J N F K N Q G I A R
F E E L I N G S G B L U E S L D
J F R S T L E S I C R E X E I
K U B E H A V I O R S T Y G R N
F L E S Y H T W O N K K N N O E
R A M O U T P E C N O C F L E S
L I F E S T Y L E R I C H A N S
```

D. ADDITIONAL ACTIVITY

General irritability, hyperexcitation, or depression
Pounding of the heart
Dryness of the throat and mouth
Impulsive behavior, emotional instability
Overpowering urge to cry, run, or hide
Inability to concentrate
Weakness or dizziness
Fatigue
Tension and keyed up alertness
Trembling and nervous tics
Intermittent anxiety
Tendency to be easily startled
High-pitched nervous laughter
Stuttering and other speech difficulties
Grinding teeth

Insomnia
Inability to sit still or physically relax
Sweating
Frequent need to urinate
Diarrhea, indigestion, queasiness, and vomiting
Migraine and other tension headaches
Premenstrual tension or missed menstrual cycles
Pain in the neck or lower back
Loss of or excessive appetite
Increased use of chemicals including tobacco, caffeine, alcohol
Nightmares
Neurotic behavior
Psychosis
Accident proneness